Parkinson's Disease and Quality of Life

Parkinson's Disease and Quality of Life has been co-published simultaneously as *Loss, Grief & Care*, Volume 8, Numbers 3/4 2000.

The *Loss, Grief & Care* Monographic "Separates"

Below is a list of "separates," which in serials librarianship means a special issue simultaneously published as a special journal issue or double-issue *and* as a "separate" hardbound monograph. (This is a format which we also call a "DocuSerial")

"Separates" are published because specialized libraries or professionals may wish to purchase a specific thematic issue by itself in a format which can be separately cataloged and shelved, as opposed to purchasing the journal on an on-going basis. Faculty members may also more easily consider a "separate" for classroom adoption.

"Separates" are carefully classified separately with the major book jobbers so that the journal tie-in can be noted on new book order slips to avoid duplicate purchasing.

You may wish to visit Haworth's website at . . .

http://www.haworthpressinc.com

. . . to search our online catalog for complete tables of contents of these separates and related publications.

You may also call 1-800-HAWORTH (outside US/Canada: 607-722-5857), or Fax 1-800-895-0582 (outside US/Canada: 607-771-0012), or e-mail at:

getinfo@haworthpressinc.com

Parkinson's Disease and Quality of Life, edited by Lucien Côté et al. (Vol. 8, No. 3/4, 2000). *Examines current research and issues of Parkinson's Disease, including health care, depression, and physician-patient relationships in order to improve the quality of life for people suffering from this long-term illness.*

After Stroke: Enhancing Quality of Life, Wallace Sife, PhD (Vol. 8, No. 1/2, 1998). *Includes the latest developments in the treatment for stroke.*

Dermatology and Person-Threatening Illness: The Patient, the Family, the Staff, edited by Robert R. Walther, MD, FACP, Agnes Beachman, RN, and Iona H. Ginsburg, MD (Vol. 7, No. 3/4, 1996). *"Very well-researched and tabulated; the references are excellent. The abstracting bibliography will make a useful reference guide to all workers involved with patients having dermatological disorders, especially where psychosocial considerations are necessary." (Palliative Medicine)*

Perspectives on Life-Threatening Illness for Allied Health Professionals, edited by Leslie M. Thompson, PhD, John G. Bruhn, PhD, Austin H. Kutscher, DDS, Barbara E. Neuhaus, EdD, OTR, F. David Cordova, EdD, and Daniel J. Cherico, PhD, MPH (Vol. 7, No. 1/2, 1993). *"Thoroughly explores the many facets and the critical reality of the breakdown and oversights within the health care delivery system. . . . An invaluable resource for administrators, policymakers, educators, and health care service providers of all capacities." (Ben E. Dickerson, PhD, Director, Institute of Gerontological Studies, Baylor University)*

Recreation, Leisure and Chronic Illness: Therapeutic Rehabilitation as Intervention in Health Care, Miriam P. Lahey, PhD, Robin Kunstler, RED, Arnold H. Grossman, PhD, Frances Daly, MS, Stuart Waldman, MS, and Fred Schwartz (Vol. 6, No. 4, 1993). *"A wonderful, positive statement about life and the roles leisure, therapeutic recreation, and play have in affirming life even in the midst of death, chronic illness, and life-threatening conditions.. . . . Must reading for educators, professionals, and students of all disciplines dealing with these very special populations." (Kathleen N. Nitschelm, MEd, CTRS, Therapeutic Recreation Consultant/Educator, New York City)*

The Physician and Hospice Care: Roles, Attitudes, and Issues, edited by Wilma Bulkin, MD, James E. Cimino, MD, David I. Wollner, MD, Austin H. Kutscher, DDS, Samuel C. Klagsbrun, MD, Terry Kinzel, MD, and Patrice M. O'Conner, RN, MA (Vol. 6, No. 2/3, 1993). *"Serves . . . to inform those who are planning to work in . . . hospice care about the main problems they will face; and as reiteration for those already involved in a hospice program." (Annals of Oncology)*

The Thanatology Community and the Needs of the Movement, edited by Elizabeth J. Clark, PhD, MSW

(Vol. 6, No. 1, 1992). *"Aims to increase the interest and awareness of thanatology and our approach to this important aspect of care. (Cancer Forum)*

Psychosocial Aspects of Narcolepsy, edited by Meeta Goswami, PhD, MPH, Charles P. Pollak, MD, Felissa L. Cohen, RN, PhD, Michael J. Thorpy, MD, Neil B. Kavey, MD, and Austin H. Kutscher, DDS (Vol. 5, No. 3/4, 1992). *"Focuses on the impact narcolepsy has on a person's day-to-day life. It addresses the diagnosis, treatment, and management of narcolepsy with particular emphasis on psychological and social aspects of care."* (Sci Tech Book News)

Psychosocial Aspects of End-Stage Renal Disease: Issues of Our Times, edited by Mark A. Hardy, John Kiernan, Austin Kutscher, Lynn Cahill, Alan I. Benevenisty (Vol. 5, No. 1/2, 1991). *"Renal disease patients, their families, and caregivers will benefit from this manual which explains the effects of this long-term illness, the psychosocial aspects involved, ethical issues related to treatment, and staff/patient perspectives."* (Senior News)

Muscular Dystrophy and Other Neuromuscular Diseases: Psychosocial Issues, edited by Leon I. Charash, Robert E. Lovelace, MD, FRCP, Claire F. Leach, Austin Kutscher, DDS, Rabbi Jacob Goldberg, and David Price Roye, Jr., MD (Vol. 4, No. 3/4, 1991). *"Helpful to professionals who assist persons with neuromuscular disorders to help them and their families to adapt to a changing lifestyle."* (Senior News)

Nursing Education in Thanatology: A Curriculum Continuum, edited by Florence E. Selder, RN, PhD, Virginia W. Barrett, RN, MEd, Marilyn M. Rawnsley, PhD, Austin H. Kutscher, DDS, Carole A. Lambert, MPA, RN, Marcia Fishman, RN, and Mary Kachoyeanos, RN, EdD (Vol. 4, No. 1/2, 1991). *"Offers nurses and other health professionals a practical and theoretical guide to compassionate care of patients and their families during the process of dying."* (Constance Captain, PhD, RN, Associate Chief of Nursing Research, Audie Murphy Memorial VA Hospital, San Antonio, Texas)

Genetic Disease: The Unwanted Inheritance, edited by John D. Rainer, Sylvia P. Rubin, Jack E. Maidman, Austin H. Kutscher, Michael K. Bartalos, Kwame Anyane-Yeboa, Phyllis Taterka, and Joanne Malin (Vol. 3, No. 3/4, 1989). *Here is a comprehensive book on the challenges faced by persons and families who find themselves affected by genetic disease and/or birth defects.*

Professional Burnout in Medicine and the Helping Professions, edited by D. Thomas Wessells, Jr., EdD, Austin H. Kutscher, DDS, Irene B. Seeland, MD, Florence E. Selder, PhD, RN, Daniel J. Cherico, PhD, and Elizabeth J. Clark, PhD, ACSW (Vol. 3, No. 1/2, 1989). *"An excellent source of basic information that summarizes the current state of research and theory development concerning health care-related stress and burnout."* (Oncology Nursing Forum)

Dying and Disabled Children: Dealing with Loss and Grief, edited by Harold M. Dick, MD, David Price Roye, Jr., MD, Penelope R. Buschman, RN, Austin H. Kutscher, DDS, Boris Rubinstein, MD, MPH, and Frances K. Forstenzer, LCSW (Vol. 2, No. 3/4, 1989). *"A valuable guide to helping professionals, as well as providing selected supplemental reading for particular clients who are learning to cope with loss."* (Residential Treatment of Children & Youth)

Thanatology Curriculum-Medicine, edited by Robert DeBellis, MD, Eric R. Marcus, MD, Austin H. Kutscher, DDS, Samuel C. Klagsbrun, MD, Irene B. Seeland, and David W. Preven, MD (Vol. 2, No. 1/2, 1998). *This compassionate volume focuses on the development of the thanatology curriculum-teaching caregivers who are just beginning their professional lives to be adequately prepared to deal appropriately with dying patients and their families and to cope with the personal toll exacted by this aspect of medical practice.*

Psychosocial Aspects of Chemotherapy in Cancer Care: The Patient, Family, and Staff, edited by Robert DeBellis, MD, George A. Hyman, MD, Irene B. Seeland, MD, Austin H. Kutscher, DDS, Alison Kimberg, RN, BSN, Mary-Ellen Siegel, MSW, ACSW, and Lillian G. Kutscher (Vol. 1, No. 3/4, 1987). *"Includes a remarkable range of commentaries and information on these issues by thoughtful and experienced clinicians."* (Cancer Forum)

Suffering: Psychological and Social Aspects in Loss, Grief, and Care, edited by Robert DeBellis, MD, Eric R. Marcus, MD, Austin H. Kutscher, DDS, Carole Smith Torres, CAC, Virginia Barrett, RN, MEd, and Mary-Ellen Siegel, MSW, ACSW (Vol. 1, No. 1/2, 1986). *Learn to understand, cope with, and even overcome-and help others overcome-emotional and physical suffering.*

Parkinson's Disease and Quality of Life

Lucien Côté
Lola L. Sprinzeles
Robin Elliott
Austin H. Kutscher
Editors

Parkinson's Disease and Quality of Life has been co-published simultaneously as *Loss, Grief & Care*, Volume 8, Numbers 3/4 2000.

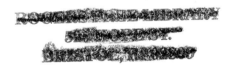

The Haworth Press, Inc.
New York • London • Oxford

Parkinson's Disease and Quality of Life has been co-published simultaneously as *Loss, Grief & Care*, Volume 8, Numbers 3/4 2000.

The development, preparation, and publication of this work has been undertaken with great care. However, the publisher, employees, editors, and agents of The Haworth Press and all imprints of The Haworth Press, Inc., including The Haworth Medical Press and Pharmaceutical Products Press, are not responsible for any errors contained herein or for consequences that may ensue from use of materials or information contained in this work. Opinions expressed by the author(s) are not necessarily those of The Haworth Press, Inc.

The Haworth Press, Inc., 10 Alice Street, Binghamton, NY 13904-1580 USA

Cover design by Thomas J. Mayshock Jr.

Library of Congress Cataloging-in-Publication Data

Parkinson's Disease and Quality of Life / Lucien Côté ... [et al.] editors.
     p. cm.
    "Parkinson's disease and quality of Life has been co-published simultaneously as Loss, grief & care, Volume 8, numbers 3/4, 2000."
    Includes bibliographical references and index.
    ISBN 0-7890-0763-0 (alk. paper).–ISBN 0-7890-0810-6 (alk. paper)
    1. Parkinson's disease. 2. Quality of Life. I. Côté, Lucien A. II. Loss, grief & care. vol. 8, no. 3-4, 1998.
RC382.P259 2000
616.8'33–dc21   00-028034

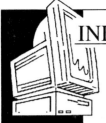

INDEXING & ABSTRACTING

Contributions to this publication are selectively indexed or abstracted in print, electronic, online, or CD-ROM version(s) of the reference tools and information services listed below. This list is current as of the copyright date of this publication. See the end of this section for additional notes.

- *Abstracts of Research in Pastoral Care & Counseling*
- *Academic Abstracts/CD-ROM*
- *AgeInfo CD-Rom*
- *Applied Social Sciences Index & Abstracts (ASSIA) (Online: ASSI via Data-Star) (CDRom: ASSIA Plus)*
- *BUBL Information Service. An Internet-based Information Service for the UK higher education community <URL:http:www.bubl.ac.uk/>*
- *CINAHL (Cumulative Index to Nursing & Allied Health Literature), in print, also on CD-ROM from CD PLUS, EBSCO, and SilverPlatter, and online from CDP Online (formerly BRS), Data-Star, and PaperChase. (Support materials include Subject Heading List, Database Search Guide, and instructional video)*
- *CNPIEC Reference Guide: Chinese National Directory of Foreign Periodicals*
- *Communication Abstracts*
- *Family Studies Database (online and CD/ROM)*
- *Health Source: Indexing & Abstracting of 160 selected health related journals, updated monthly*
- *Health Source Plus: expanded version of "Health Source" to be released shortly*
- *IBZ International Bibliography of Periodical Literature*
- *Leeds Medical Information*
- *Mental Health Abstracts (online through DIALOG)*
- *New Literature on Old Age*
- *Referativnyi Zhurnal (Abstracts Journal of the All-Russian Institute of Scientific and Technical Information)*

(continued)

- *Sage Family Studies Abstracts (SFSA)*
- *Sapient Health Network*
- *Social Planning/Policy & Development Abstracts (SOPODA)*
- *Social Work Abstracts*
- *Sociological Abstracts (SA)*

Special Bibliographic Notes related to special journal issues (separates) and indexing/abstracting:

- indexing/abstracting services in this list will also cover material in any "separate" that is co-published simultaneously with Haworth's special thematic journal issue or DocuSerial. Indexing/abstracting usually covers material at the article/chapter level.
- monographic co-editions are intended for either non-subscribers or libraries which intend to purchase a second copy for their circulating collections.
- monographic co-editions are reported to all jobbers/wholesalers/approval plans. The source journal is listed as the "series" to assist the prevention of duplicate purchasing in the same manner utilized for books-in-series.
- to facilitate user/access services all indexing/abstracting services are encouraged to utilize the co-indexing entry note indicated at the bottom of the first page of each article/chapter/contribution.
- this is intended to assist a library user of any reference tool (whether print, electronic, online, or CD-ROM) to locate the monographic version if the library has purchased this version but not a subscription to the source journal.
- individual articles/chapters in any Haworth publication are also available through the Haworth Document Delivery Service (HDDS).

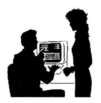

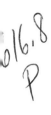

Parkinson's Disease
and Quality of Life

CONTENTS

The American Institute of Life-Threatening Illness and Loss, the Parkinson's Disease Foundation, and the editors acknowledge their appreciation for the editorial asistance of Danielle Green.

Shortness of Breath
Among Persons with Parkinson's Disease

Norma M. T. Braun

Data for the pulmonary causes of shortness of breath (SOB) in Parkinson's disease is mostly lacking. An informal canvas of a group of neurologists to determine the major causes of morbidity and mortality in this group of patients will often indicate either pneumonia or urosepsis. One of the major causes of death is pneumonia. There are changes in the breathing pattern of Parkinson's disease patients. Whether this alteration in breathing pattern predisposes to pneumonia is wholly unknown. Dysphagia resulting in aspiration pneumonia is another cause of pulmonary compromise. Dyspnea is shortness of breath or a sense of insufficient air intake for the task. This restricts life. It is a symptom which is difficult to quantify because each patient has his or her own threshold or perception of difficulty in breathing.

Since Parkinson's is frequently a disease of aging, many patients may also have asthma, bronchitis, emphysema, or heart disease, especially if they were smokers in the past. These factors add to the respiratory load. Enumerated here are some of the features which contribute to dyspnea in Parkinson's patients who do not have additional major primary cardiac or pulmonary diseases. Breathing control functions in a closed loop system. Breathing is a fundamental function of respiratory drive from the central nervous system with many inputs and feedback to the brain which then alters the output in response. Shallow patterns of breathing result in reducing the level of oxygenation; the brain does not tolerate lack of oxygen.

In addition, patients with Parkinson's disease often have sleep disturbance, due either to the primary disease or to its treatment. This results in daytime

Norma M. T. Braun, MD, PC, is affiliated with St. Luke's-Roosevelt Hospital Center, Physician's Office, 1090 Amsterdam Avenue, New York, NY 10025.

[Haworth co-indexing entry note]: "Shortness of Breath Among Persons with Parkinson's Disease." Braun, Norma M.T.. Co-published simultaneously in *Loss, Grief & Care* (The Haworth Press, Inc.) Vol. 8, No. 3/4, 2000, pp. 1-5; and: *Parkinson's Disease and Quality of Life* (ed: Côté et al.) The Haworth Press, Inc., 2000, pp. 1-5. Single or multiple copies of this article are available for a fee from The Haworth Document Delivery Service [1-800-342-9678, 9:00 a.m. - 5:00 p.m. (EST). E-mail address: getinfo@ haworthpressinc.com].

dysfunction. Insomnia and frequent arousals may be due to either central or obstructive apneas, both of which can be treated. Excessive limb movements at night may also cause arousal and sleep talking or somnambulism may occur despite their usual rigidity. The paradox is that less movement in bed due to rigidity may itself result in arousals. When the sleep disorder is identified and treated, daytime sleepiness and function can be much improved.

It would also be appropriate to focus on dysynchronous activity of upper airway and respiratory muscles which can follow endotracheal intubation and which may first become clinically manifest after hip fracture repair, which is a common occurrence due to their predisposition to falls. Surgical correction is usually necessary and patients are intubated for anesthesia. Following intubation dysphagia may worsen, and when not recognized, aspiration pneumonia can follow. Resolution of the aspiration pneumonia is slow due to a very weak cough. This is the major reason why patients may require reintubation or may remain intubated, prolonging the time of hospitalization and recovery.

The following is a brief overview of the consequences of Parkinson's disease on pulmonary function, respiratory rhythm, the respiratory muscles, and gas exchange. The respiratory muscles are bradykinetic and are slower in their activation to contraction. We can measure the ability to take a great big breath and the rate at which breathing is accomplished in the pulmonary function lab. This is respiratory gymnastics. The vital capacity is often reduced, and the ability to generate air flow is reduced. There appears to be increased airflow resistance, due either to intrinsic alteration of airways tone from cholinergic influences and/or the inability to generate a rapid velocity of muscle contraction to produce flow. Chest wall mechanical elastic recoil force is markedly reduced which also limits the capacity to generate air flow. The ability to move air quickly, repeatedly, or the maximum voluntary ventilation, is markedly attenuated, and the total amount of breathing per unit time, the minute ventilation, may be reduced. Thus the rigid chest/muscle system causes the shallow pattern which feeds back to the brain to adapt a more rapid breathing cycle. Parkinson's disease patients also sigh much less. Sighs are maximal slow inspirations and normally reduce the stiffness of the lungs and chest cage and increase the flexibility of the rib cage joints. As patients become dyspneic they become less active which further deconditions them.

Upper airway caliber is also restricted by the head flexed diameter. The rib cage is also restricted by the bent forward position, since it is now sitting on the pelvic brim. The muscles become fore-shortened and therefore cannot shorten more and thus contract with less force. Less force results in weak coughs. Parkinson's disease patients are thus loaded from both outside and inside with an altered respiratory drive. The return to more normal function with medication reduces or abolishes dyspnea which, by vida infra, supports the hypothesis that these ventilatory derangements are due to the effect of Parkinson's disease on upper airway and respiratory muscles.

The consequence of the disturbances in breathing pattern is an alteration in blood gas exchange. This pattern of breathing causes a maldistribution of air to blood flow which results in reducing arterial oxygen tension. If there is primary lung disease, this worsens. Elevation of carbon dioxide (pCO_2) levels generally does not occur until very late in the course of this disease. Maybe part of the reason why these patients are not referred for respiratory evaluation until late is that they don't complain until they are dyspneic with daily activities or at rest. The reason is that the amount of air one needs to breathe for quiet living is five percent of maximum capacity. So if one only needs five cents out of every dollar to spend for everyday living it requires a lot of loss before one realizes that one is bankrupt. As patients become more bradykinetic they do less and less, and may never exceed their reduced capacity, therefore, they are much worse before they complain. If the patient doesn't complain the doctor may not heed the respiratory system.

This is one of the things that happen during the flow/volume loop of a normal person. The amount of air that can be inhaled is breathed in to a very rapid peak at a maximal flow rate, until the lungs are filled when flow rates decline. The whole system then recoils aided by a large group of expiratory muscles which push all the air out. The slope of the expiratory curve is a function of airway caliber, which decreases with reducing lung volume. This is a very predictable relationship. Patient data are compared to a standard-normal, from which the patient's deviation is measured.

Patients with associated dystonic adduction of vocal cords, that is when the vocal cords are closing on inspiration, can actually develop stridor, causing interruptions in the flow volume curve. Extremely low flow rates do not generate stridor. Interruption of airflow due to closure of the upper airways from spasms or tremor cause other patterns. Unfortunately we can't easily discriminate the spasm or tremor from the upper airways from the same process occurring from the respiratory muscles. One of the ways to separate the upper airways from the respiratory muscles is to videofluoroscope them. Videofluoroscopy of the chest wall diaphragm may allow visualization of tremors of both. There may also be dysynchrony between the two sides in the same subject. Tremors may be on inspiration or expiration or both with tremendous variation. Each patient has his/her own particular contour, and each effort may be different. Unless one examines all the patterns the abnormality may be missed. (The technician may decide it is a technically bad tracing, and discard it). Quiet breathing may be normal but attempts at increasing breathing rates may expose the variable breathing patterns. Normally one can repeat a rapid breathing maneuver uniformly until fatigue, but these patients have marked variation of each tidal breath, with hesitations.

Some patients will grunt either on inspiration or on expiration. They could be so soft that they are not noted unless they're noisy enough to make family members bring it to the physician's attention. These abnormal respiratory patterns are associated with the sensation of dyspnea. Medication for Parkinson's disease can improve or reduce or abolish the dyspnea.

We looked at 25 Parkinson's disease patients who complained of dyspnea as a primary complaint, of whom 14 had changes that we could measure. Most of these patients had severe on-off phenomenon which is why they were being referred. Their symptom of dyspnea was always worst at their off period, with frequencies roughly from a few per day to several per week. The duration of their symptoms varied from minutes to hours, which were often relieved or alleviated by dopaminergic agents. There were 15 men and 10 women. The mean age was 58 years with a range of 31 to 79. The duration of Parkinsonism was about eleven years with a range from 4 to 22 years. Length of treatment with L-dopa was about nine years but again with a wide range; all but one were currently on L-dopa drugs. Parkinson's disease score when on drugs was 87 mean, with a wide range; and when off the mean was 47, a significant difference. They had axial bradykinesia on physical examination. Respiratory function during off periods tended to be with a shallow breathing pattern with poor excursions of their chest wall and abdomen, indicating both chest cage and diaphragmatic rigidity. A restricted vital capacity is the consequence. Their breathing frequencies when off tended to be much more rapid, from 25 to 100 percent over their baseline value. An Xray taken during an off period tends to appear to be on expiration. The radiologist will interpret it as a poor inspiratory effort. Blood gases may be normal or abnormal depending upon how long that pattern has been present. One patient allowed us to place both esophageal and gastric balloons so we could directly measure the rate of force of contraction, the amount of pressure developed and the ratio of inspiratory time to total ventilatory time. He had a pre-Sinemet vital capacity of 3.5 liters, Sinemet increased it to 4.5 liters. Also minute ventilation increased after Sinemet and breathing frequencies fall because breaths are now deeper. Normal inspiratory time (T_I) is 0. 3 of total cycle time (T_{TOT}). Parkinson's disease patients spend more time on inspiration; that is T_I may be 0.6 or more. After Sinemet T_I, shortens towards normal but may not be restored to the 0.3 ratio. Transdiaphragmatic pressures, measured from the esophageal and gastric balloons, can double after Sinemet. Are these weak muscles, or only bradykinetic muscles? Maximum expiratory pressure is essential for coughing, and clearing airways. Maximum expiratory pressures can double after medication, turning an ineffective cough to an effective, protective one. A single dose of 20/200 L-dopa can double the cough force. Some patients respond quickly and others much more slowly, possibly due to variable GI rates of absorption. The patients we studied behaved in the same way: All respiratory function was depressed when they were off and all improved after Sinemet, with individuation of the degree of change in each patient.

In summary, respiratory function is a motor act that may be affected in Parkinson's disease. We see changes in the frequency and severity of brady-kinesia and variation in responsiveness to drugs. Fluctuations in respiratory function are frequent, may be complicated by sleep disorder and appear to be part of the clinical oscillations. Dyspnea can be from upper airway and chest/diaphragm dysynchrony and when off will respond to therapy but rarely returns completely to normal. The partial reversibility of bradykinesia associated with dyspnea relief suggests that the altered pattern of muscular contractions causes dyspnea.

REFERENCES

Braun, NMU. Spirometry & Flow Volume Loops. Chapter 10, pp. 108-116. IN: Neurologic Disorders of the Larynx. Eds. A. Blitzer, M. Brin, C. Sasahi, K. Harris. Thieme Medical Publishers, Inc. NY, 1992.

Ilson, J., Braun, NMT., Fahn, S. Respiratory Fluctuations in Parkinson's Disease. Neurology 1983; 33 (Suppl.2): 113, Abs.

Accessing Benefits
for Parkinson's Patients

Judith Brickman

Before describing some of the specific benefits available to assist persons with Parkinson's disease, I would like to give you some suggestions about accessing these benefits for patients and their families. They may seem elementary, but they do work.

(1) When calling an agency, have something to do while waiting. When talking to answering machines there is a temptation to hang up. But remember, if you hang up, whenever you call back it's going to be the same. Take a crossword puzzle, knitting or something else to do.

(2) When one does get through to somebody, obtain their name and write it down. Write it in gold. Do not lose it. It is really important to know to whom you are speaking.

(3) When you do get somebody on the phone, have all the material available that will be needed. Agency staff members don't have any more time or patience than you do.

(4) If you send something in the mail when applying for any benefits, make copies to keep and send these by registered mail. It's worth spending a little more money so that somebody can't say, "We never got it from you."

(5) Be persistent in following through, but don't call too soon. If somebody tells you it will take approximately four weeks, you're not going to accomplish anything by calling in two weeks. You're just going to get on the wrong side of somebody who you may yet need. However, do not wait six weeks to call. If you don't hear in four weeks, call.

Judith Brickman, CSW, is Coordinator, Residency and Nursing Home Affairs, New York City Department for the Aging, New York, NY.

[Haworth co-indexing entry note]: "Accessing Benefits for Parkinson's Patients." Brickman, Judith. Co-published simultaneously in *Loss, Grief & Care* (The Haworth Press, Inc.) Vol. 8, No. 3/4, 2000, pp. 7-9; and: *Parkinson's Disease and Quality of Life* (ed: Côté et al.) The Haworth Press, Inc., 2000, pp. 7-9. Single or multiple copies of this article are available for a fee from The Haworth Document Delivery Service [1-800-342-9678, 9:00 a.m. - 5:00 p.m. (EST). E-mail address: getinfo@haworthpressinc.com].

(6) What you may have to do is go up the ladder. If you find, after two or three conversations with the person you are speaking to that you are not successful, ask for their supervisor. Go all the way to the top.

(7) It may not always be easy, but courtesy really does help. Now that ways to access benefits have been discussed these are descriptions of some specific programs.

    (a) *Medicare.* Medicare is a benefit for those over 65 but, if you are younger and have received disability benefits for 24 months or more, then you also qualify for Medicare. Medicare has Part A and Part B. Part A will pay for hospitals and nursing home care, if certain criteria are met, and hospice. Part B will pay for doctors' bills, medical equipment, and the like. The current telephone number is 1-800/772-1213 to learn more about Medicare.

    (b) *Social Security.* Social Security is a benefit which you are entitled to if you've worked under Social Security. The amount varies according to what you have earned. In 1995, the amount of increase was the second lowest COLA–cost of living allowance raise in Social Security's history. To obtain more information about Social Security call 1-800/722-1213.

    (c) *Veterans Benefits.* Many people do not realize there are Veterans' benefits and don't try to access those to which they are entitled such as hospitalization and Nursing Home coverage. The telephone number to access Veterans Administration benefits is 212/620-6901.

    (d) *Medicaid.* Medicaid is a benefit which is based on financial need rather than age. Eligibility is determined on the basis of income and resources. One should be aware that different types of Medicaid assistance have different requirements. If you are found ineligible for Medicaid Home Care, you may still qualify for Medicaid Nursing Home coverage and vice versa. In addition to Home Care and Nursing Homes, Medicaid covers hospitals, physicians, laboratory bills, medication, medical equipment and transportation for medical appointments and other medical related expenses. For more information about Medicaid, call the HRA information line, (718) 291-1900.

    (e) *Transportation.* Transportation is a significant problem for those with Parkinson's disease. In New York City, there is a half-fare program for those over 65 and it's very simple. All you have to do is show a Medicare card. For those under 65 who are disabled, the application process is slightly different. There are also two other programs in New York City. One of them is sponsored by the subway system and its called Access-a-Ride. It is not an age-based program but rather for anybody who is handicapped or has some kind of disability. The Access-a-Ride telephone number is (718) 694-3581. One problem with the Access-a-Ride program is that there may be more people who need rides than there are rides available. Registering with Access-a-Ride takes about four or five weeks. Once it's approved you can call in the beginning of the month to schedule regular appointments, or a few days before for one-time trips. Access-a-Ride will not provide transportation from one borough to another. For people over 60, the Department for the Aging has transportation programs throughout the five boroughs. In order to obtain information about specific areas call the Department's Information and Referral unit at (212) 442-1000.

There are many additional benefits and entitlements available to people with Parkinson's disease. Please call the Parkinson's Foundation or the Department for the Aging for further information.

Physician and Patients
in Managing Parkinson's Disease

Mitchell F. Brin

INTRODUCTION

An essential component of a physician-patient relationship is an adequate ability for the physician to communicate with the patient, and also for the patient to relay their current symptomatology directly to the physician. This report will outline some of the limitations that are problematic as a function of the current health care system. In addition, I will make some recommendations on how physicians and patients can better communicate in an effort to improve overall patient care.

TREATING PATIENTS IN THE CURRENT MEDICAL ERA

In the past, physicians had the luxury of spending a considerable amount of time with patients in the office in a setting where one had very few time or financial constraints. In the current era of the shrinking health care dollar, and also with increased demands put upon the medical system, it is crucial to identify ways to utilize the scarcest and most precious resource: time.

Most physicians are addressing an increase in the size of their patient population. Furthermore, the aging population has more complex medical problems. Physicians are under fire with more paperwork and documentation, and this is hampered by limitations on reimbursement which would

Mitchell F. Brin, MD, is Associate Professor of Neurology and Co-Director, Movement Disorder Center, The Mount Sinai Medical Center, New York, NY 10029-6574.

[Haworth co-indexing entry note]: "Physician and Patients in Managing Parkinson's Disease." Brin, Mitchell F. Co-published simultaneously in *Loss, Grief & Care* (The Haworth Press, Inc.) Vol. 8, No. 3/4, 2000, pp. 11-13; and: *Parkinson's Disease and Quality of Life* (ed: Côté et al.) The Haworth Press, Inc., 2000, pp. 11-13. Single or multiple copies of this article are available for a fee from The Haworth Document Delivery Service [1-800-342-9678, 9:00 a.m. - 5:00 p.m. (EST). E-mail address: getinfo@haworthpress inc.com].

normally permit physicians to obtain additional resources. The problems are further complicated by the trend towards managed care sweeping across the country, constantly modifying access to medical care.

The following are some guidelines addressed to patients to help them prepare for a visit to the doctor. These ideas are designed to make the visit more efficient and satisfactory for both the patient and the doctor.

By adhering to these fundamental concepts, the office visit will proceed in a more orderly and smooth fashion, and permit the treating physician to obtain important historical and examination information to synthesize a treatment plan and shepherd patients through their disease.

VISITING THE DOCTOR'S OFFICE

Preparing

Patients should prepare to come to the doctor's office. It will help make the visit more efficient for both you and your physician. Thinking about these things in advance will enable you and the doctor to focus on the issues that are important to you. Doctors typically ask similar questions at each visit. Usually these are:

1. Which medications are you currently taking?
2. What was the impact of the last change in your medication program?
3. Are there any new symptoms?
4. Do you have any new medical problems?
5. Do you have any additional questions?

At this point the doctor will probably perform an examination, answer your questions, develop a treatment plan, discuss the new treatment plan, and send you on your way.

Therefore, it is critical you provide information early on in the office consultation. When preparing to discuss these issues *prior to* coming to the office, you will also need to reflect on symptoms and signs. Here are some suggestions to guide your reflections.

1. How often do symptoms occur? Are symptoms occasional or frequent?
2. With respect to episodes or symptoms, what occurs and when?

You will need to describe the impact of any drug changes on overall management of the disease and describe and summarize the symptoms. In order to do this effectively, it would be helpful to learn the fundamental language and "lingo" of Parkinson's disease. Descriptive terms such as "on," "off," "wearing off," "dyskinesia," "dystonia," "freezing," "sudden on-off" need to be mastered.

You should bring a written list of all medications, including non-PD medications, you are taking to the office visit. The list should include the time of each dose, the amount taken at each time, and the amount of medication in each pill. The doctor will compare this information with the information in the medical record to see if there are any unexpected changes since the last visit. It is also helpful if you can bring a list of any new general medical events, new Parkinson's disease specific events, and the results of tests and office visits with other physicians that may have occurred since the last visit with your Parkinson doctor. It is useful to jot down any changes that have occurred in disease symptoms since the last medication change and list any side effects since the last visit.

At the Visit

During the office visit, ask all of your questions. Listen very carefully when the doctor makes recommendations. Ask questions to clarify these recommendations and other issues. Write down the answers. Sometimes, after leaving the doctor's office, a patient will wonder "what did he just tell me," or "what am I suppose to do now." The best time to ask these questions is in the office. Unless your doctor is told that you do not understand, your doctor will not be able to help you.

Sometimes there may be medical forms or disability forms you need the doctor to complete, or other such tasks. These should be presented to the physician at the *beginning* of the office visit so that the doctor may complete them at the appropriate times during the office visit.

As the visit nears a close, final questions should be asked and any loose ends should be tied up.

The Final Gift:
Autopsy and Brain Donation

Susan Calne

Evidence from as far back as two thousand years before Christ shows that man has had a continuing curiosity about how the brain works and has wanted to look inside it. Hippocrates, in 400 B.C., wrote a tract on epilepsy that is regarded even by some in the twentieth century as the best discussion of the brain.

It was not until the late nineteenth century that the general public began to lose its aversion to doctors examining the insides of dead bodies. Literature is littered with grave robbers and characters like the idealistic Dr. Lydgate in Middlemarch who was roundly censured by the inhabitants of the town because he cut open dead bodies at the infirmary. He was determined to find the cure for cholera and typhus.

Modern neuropathology had its beginnings in Germany at the end of the nineteenth century. The physicians of the time may have had less difficulty with the public than Dr. Lydgate had because they were now beginning to effect a positive change in peoples' health instead of just offering a bottle of "tonic" and being at the bedside when the patient expired. They were beginning to inspire trust. The most notable neuropathologist was Alois Alzheimer who began his training in Frankfurt and while there began his association with Franz Nissl (Haymaker, W. S., 1970). These men developed histological stains that revolutionized the way researchers could look at tissue.

Susan Calne, RN, is Clinical Coordinator, Neurodegenerative Disorders Centre, Vancouver Hospital and Health Sciences Centre, The University of British Columbia, Vancouver, British Columbia, Canada.

The author thanks Drs. Pat McGeer and Tom Beech for advice and help preparing this paper. The author acknowledges the support of The Parkinson Foundation of Canada, The Dystonia Medical Research Foundation and the National Parkinson Foundation (Miami).

[Haworth co-indexing entry note]: "The Final Gift: Autopsy and Brain Donation." Calne, Susan. Co-published simultaneously in Loss, Grief & Care (The Haworth Press, Inc.) Vol. 8, No. 3/4, 2000, pp. 15-20; and: Parkinson's Disease and Quality of Life (ed: Côté et al.) The Haworth Press, Inc., 2000, pp. 15-20. Single or multiple copies of this article are available for a fee from The Haworth Document Delivery Service [1-800-342-9678, 9:00 a.m. - 5:00 p.m. (EST). E-mail address: getinfo@haworthpressinc.com].

Until Charcot's appointment as Professor of Pathological Anatomy in Paris in 1857, studies on the brain had largely been anatomical. Neurochemistry was more dependent on the parallel evolution of new technical advances in the laboratories of general chemists and the understanding of quantitative analysis. The names of prominent nineteenth century neuropathologists such as Charcot, Alzheimer and Jacob are perhaps more familiar to us than those of the neurochemists because illnesses have been named after them.

Neurochemical studies related to Parkinsonism did not really begin until the turn of the twentieth century when the work of Haliburton, Elliott, Dale and Dudley began the identification of what we now know to be neurotransmitters (Haymaker, W. S. 1970). These 'messenger' chemicals transmit messages between nerve endings to allow the brain to carry out its endless, complex functions.

James Parkinson never examined a postmortem brain and the reason for the symptoms he so eloquently described eluded researchers until the early nineteen sixties when Ehringer, Hornykiewicz, and Birkmayer identified dopamine as the missing neurotransmitter in Parkinsonism (Ehringer, H. et al. 1960).

The loss of the distinctive black melanin, visible to the naked eye, in the substantia nigra is evidence of the death of dopamine producing cells that results in the symptoms of Idiopathic Parkinsonism. The presence of Lewy bodies in the brains of patients dying with Parkinsonism is still regarded by some as the definitive post mortem diagnostic marker but there is an argument revolving around this as they may be present in the brains of elderly normal subjects as well as those with other neurodegenerative disorders.

These discoveries evolving over almost a century could only have been made possible with an adequate supply of brain tissue. This knowledge could not have come about through experiments on the living brain. The impact of this discovery has meant symptomatic treatment for hundreds of thousands of people with Idiopathic Parkinsonism. This type of treatment is unknown in any other neurodegenerative disorder.

Before beginning a discussion on brain retrieval for research purposes following death, it might be helpful to put the operation in context with the more readily understood procedure of autopsy. The word autopsy is from the Greek autoptos and the Oxford English dictionary defines it as a 'personal inspection: post mortem' (Latin for after death). The general public's familiarity with autopsies usually comes from television or newspapers. A coroner orders an autopsy to determine the cause and time of death in what may turn out to be a criminal case. We are all familiar with revelations of time of death, blood types, bullet wound entries, and depth of knife stabs, etc. Tragically of late, truth has been more unbelievable than fiction. An autopsy may also be ordered if the circumstances of a death are sudden, unusual or the patient has not seen a physician for a very long time.

Autopsies take place, with the permission of the next of kin, every day in major hospitals around the world, to establish the cause of death, and to provide pathological correlations with the clinical symptoms. An autopsy is an intrinsic teaching tool for physicians. The pathologist confirms, and in some cases establishes the cause of death. These autopsies are what we call diagnostic.

Modern scanning tools, biopsies, and sophisticated body fluid analyses provide a lot of the answers for physicians. However, in the area of neurology, it remains impossible to confirm many diagnoses in life because surgery is not possible and scanning tools can not provide the answers. Thus, granting permission for an autopsy following death from a neurological disorder is a gift to medical science whose value is beyond price.

Following an autopsy, the pathologist writes a detailed report both for the attending physician and as a permanent case history. The family can have access to this report but usually in a setting where a physician is present to explain it and to answer questions. In the hospital where I work, an autopsy report is never mailed to the family. If the next of kin can not return to the clinic, the report can be mailed to the family physician who can discuss it with the family.

Families may request an autopsy if they wish to be certain about the cause of death. The unwillingness of hospital staff to perform one under these circumstances, if autopsy services are available, would be disturbing.

An even greater gift to neurological science is granting permission for brain retrieval post mortem for research purposes. There is still so much to learn about the neurochemical and molecular neuropathology of the brain that can only be done with brain tissue that is retrieved specifically for this purpose.

In practice, the brain's tissues and fluids deteriorate slowly in a mortuary cold room kept at 4° C. Following death, the brain tissue will be handled in different ways depending on whether it is going to be sent to a neuropathological brain bank (there are two in the USA) or examined in a neurochemical laboratory which will most likely be adjacent to the hospital where the death takes place. For some of the chemical and molecular investigations the tissue must be retrieved within 2-4 hours.

As this century draws to a close, neuropathologists throughout the world have an ever increasing number of methods with which to examine the microscopic chemical workings of the brain. The reasons for authorizing autopsy and brain donation are more important than ever. The need now is not so much for diagnostic purposes as the changes found in the brains of people with Parkinsonism have already been described. It is more to allow molecular neuropathologists and neurochemists to try to discover what triggers the cells to die in order to establish the cause of Idiopathic Parkinsonism or other neurological disorders. At least 40 neurotransmitters have been identified. As neurons die, their neurotransmitters disappear. While these neurotransmitters have been discovered painstakingly over the twentieth century their relationship to each other and their roles in the brain is not completely understood. We know quite a lot about dopamine: glutamate may have a role in epilepsy, serotonin with migraine and depression to name just three. The McGeers' work comparing neuronal loss in the substantia nigra in Idiopathic Parkinsonism and aging involved painstaking cell counts in the substantia nigra of a normal elderly brain, a Parkinsonian brain, and a young person's brain (McGeer, P. L. et al. 1989). Jellinger has added enormously to our knowledge of the inclusion bodies, e.g., Lewy, Hirano and Marinesco. They form in the brain as the result of the degeneration of certain vulnerable populations of neurons. However, what mechanisms bring about their development and what their development contributes to the cellular and molecular pathology of Idiopathic Parkinsonism is still unknown (Jellinger, K. 1987).

These and other important discoveries that add to our understanding of Idiopathic Parkinsonism could not have been possible without the donation of tissue. For the purposes of preparing this paper, I attended the removal of a brain from one of our patients who had signed the forms with the concurrence of her husband pre mortem. Patients and families should be reassured that the procedure is dignified and quick. There can be an open casket at the funeral if the next of kin wishes. The pathologist makes an incision over the top of the head from behind one ear to the other. The skin is eased from the skull and a square section of the skull is cut and removed. The brain is gently cut away from the base of the skull, removed, weighed and put into a container on ice. The brain cavity is packed with cotton wool or tissue, the bone section is put back in place and the skin flaps stitched together. As the stitch line is through the hair, it is invisible.

There are good reasons why people with Idiopathic Parkinsonism and the related disorders, Shy Drager syndrome, progressive supranuclear palsy and, olivo-ponto-cerebellar atrophy, should consider taking steps *during their life* to authorize the donation of their brain for research purposes post mortem. Many of the investigations currently carried out need fresh tissue. This has to be removed carefully and quickly within a few hours of death. Permission is often sought from the next of kin following the death of a patient but, because of the speed of removal required, this can and does intrude on the families' immediate distress and is a major reason why physicians are reluctant to ask for research tissue. If the issue of brain donation for research or autopsy has not been discussed by the patient with the next of kin this leaves them in an agony of indecision as they do not know what the deceased's wishes were.

I have worked in the same clinic for twelve years. One of my first tasks was to help to develop a protocol for tissue retrieval with consent forms that would meet the requirements of our ethics committee. Once this was done, my role in seeking pre-mortem permission evolved such that it is now one of my major responsibilities.

I have talked about this subject with other nurses and physicians and have been impressed with the difficulty some physicians express in approaching their patients pre-mortem. It may be that physicians find it difficult to admit to their patients that they will die. The physician is supposed to heal. Neither nurses nor physicians are taught in their respective schools that their patients will die, nor that allowing a patient a 'good death' is an honorable achievement. To the newly qualified, the first death is like a body blow. This leads to an inevitable situation where we 'learn on the job' not only to deal with grief of the family but also our own; some of us manage better than others.

My experience has been that in a clinic with a stable population of patients, many of whom have been attending the clinic since it opened, the trust that has developed between the staff and the patient and family allows me to be straightforward. In a quiet setting, I tell people that I have an important issue to discuss with them. I begin by telling them that while the donation will not benefit them it will add to our knowledge so that future generations will benefit. I describe the donation as a gift as I do believe that there are few greater gifts one can give in life than to agree to autopsy, organ donation or tissue retrieval.

In twelve years, I have only had three refusals (for religious reasons). In addition, patients and families approach clinic staff independently asking to donate tissue post-mortem. Neurologists throughout the province of British Columbia collaborate whenever possible.

Once the patient has expressed interest I insist that they discuss it with their next of kin and children (if applicable). I ask them not to sign a consent form if there is dissent in the family as this will cause added unhappiness at the time of their death. Sometimes the patient is not capable of signing the forms and the next of kin can take the responsibility by signing a consent form pre-mortem. If the forms in our protocol are signed pre-mortem there is no intrusion necessary following death. Instead there is a concerted effort on the part of the family, long term care facility/ hospital, pathologist, clinic and laboratory to ensure that the retrieval takes place in order to fulfill the wishes of the patient and family. The decision has already been made. In a way, this exercise seems to distract families from their immediate grief; it gives them something to do to tide them over the first shock. If the death is at an inconvenient hour for the pathology department and retrieval is uncertain, the family can become quite determined over the need to carry out their relative's wishes.

Brains retrieved for research purposes provide valuable tissue for many researchers over many years. The fixed Brain Bank tissue is made available to researchers all over North America. Fresh tissue is used in laboratories dedicated to this work. There is an important difference between the diagnostic autopsy and tissue retrieved for research. The latter does not generate a detailed report but series of numbers, cell counts for example, and amounts of chemicals found in tissue. It is important for the next of kin to appreciate this and not expect a written report. You should be reassured that confidentiality is guaranteed at all times.

Finally, it is important to be realistic about the practicality of tissue donation. If a person has a very common illness and dies a great distance from a center for research it is more than likely that retrieval for research purposes will not take place at the time of death. This will be because all this work is funded through research grants. Tissue retrieval is expensive and with ever diminishing research funds available, researchers have to make difficult decisions about priority that may disappoint those of you wishing to contribute to scientific discovery. The answer lies in improved funding for brain research.

REFERENCES

Ehringer H, Hornykiewicz O. Verteilung Von Noradrenalin und dopamin (3-Hydroxytyramin)im Gehirn des Menschen und ihr Verhalten bei Erkrankungen des extrapyramidalen Systems. Klin Woch 1960;38:1236-1239.

Haymaker WS. The Founders of Neurology. 2nd ed. Springfield Illinois: Charles C. Thomas, 1970:5.

Jellinger K. Cytoskeletal Pathology of Parkinsonism and Aging Brain. In: Calne DB, Comi G, Crippa D, Horowski R, Trabucchi M, eds. Parkinsonism and Aging. New York: Raven Press, 1987:35-56.

McGeer PL, Itagaki S, Akiyama H, McGeer EG. Comparison of neuronal loss in Parkinson's disease and aging. In: Calne DB, Comi G, Crippa D, Horowski R, Trabucchi M, eds. Parkinsonism and Aging. New York: Raven Press, 1989:25-34.

Intimacy, Sexuality
and Idiopathic Parkinsonism:
The Uncharted Waters

Susan Calne
Rosemary Basson

There are no absolute rights and wrongs about sex and intimacy in health or in sickness. No one has all the answers. Indeed, most of us do not know the right questions! Far from being a consistent, sustained and crystal clear feature of our lives, sex is often a much more inconsistent, fluctuating and cloudier affair, but nonetheless a precious and treasured aspect of our lives. Ideally perhaps, everyone reading this paper would say that nothing in it applies to them. If that is not the case, we hope this discussion will make some of you feel less alone with your anxieties and concerns and give you the courage to begin talking about them and to seek help if you need it.

Our aim is to describe the common sexual difficulties couples living with Parkinson's disease experience, to try to give some explanations, and more importantly, to mention the kind of help that is available.

Information about sex often starts in the school yard. If we are lucky our parents fill in the gaps. Some of us remember blushing unmarried biology teachers doing their best. A few of us only have found out what it was all

Susan Calne, RN, is Clinical Coordinator, Neurodegenerative Disorders Centre, University of British Columbia, Vancouver, British Columbia, Canada. Rosemary Basson, MD, is Clinical Assistant Professor, Sexual Medicine Clinic, University of British Columbia, Vancouver, British Columbia, Canada.

Susan Calne acknowledges the support of The Parkinson Foundation of Canada, The National Parkinson Foundation (Miami) and The Dystonia Medical Research Foundation.

[Haworth co-indexing entry note]: "Intimacy, Sexuality and Idiopathic Parkinsonism: The Uncharted Waters." Calne, Susan, and Rosemary Basson. Co-published simultaneously in *Loss, Grief & Care* (The Haworth Press, Inc.) Vol. 8, No. 3/4, 2000, pp. 21-27; and: *Parkinson's Disease and Quality of Life* (ed: Côté et al.) The Haworth Press, Inc., 2000, pp. 21-27. Single or multiple copies of this article are available for a fee from The Haworth Document Delivery Service [1-800-342-9678, 9:00 a.m. - 5:00 p.m. (EST). E-mail address: getinfo@haworthpressinc.com].

21

about as it was happening for the first time. Since Masters and Johnson brought sex into the public domain in the '60s, information has become available through two main sources. The first is the medical profession, be it physicians or psychologists reporting on their own patients' problems or conducting surveys of sexual concerns of people not identifying themselves as patients. The second is the media, television documentaries or talk shows, magazine articles and books produced by people of extremely mixed knowledge and skills. Information from the first may be too clinical, not to mention difficult to access, and from the second unrealistic and untested. Both may leave us feeling inadequate. An exception is the recently published *Sex, Love, and Chronic Illness* by Lucite Carlton, the widow of a Parkinsonian (Carlton, L. 1994).

Data about intimacy, sexuality, and Idiopathic Parkinsonism (Parkinsonism IP) are thin on the ground (Brown, R. G. et al. 1990; Lipe, H. et al. 1990). What is known, to those of us counseling patients and their partners, is that problems exist that far exceed those of simple mechanical difficulties that one might expect to accompany a decrease in mobility. So much depends on the self esteem of the individual and strength and state of a couple's emotional and physical relationship before a chronic illness intervenes. If a couple's sex life was not satisfactory before diagnosis, it will not improve without help when they have to adjust to a chronic illness at the same time. If the relationship has been happy and healthy, there is no reason why it should not continue this way for a long time. If there are physical problems arising from the changes in the way that sexual organs function, or from difficulties moving in bed, these can be addressed as necessary.

The period of adjustment to a chronic illness such as Parkinsonism takes time and some will manage better than others. It is not only sex that is uncharted; many people will live with this condition for twenty years. Everyone is different and so it is difficult to measure oneself against the progression and symptoms of someone else with the condition. At times, a person may feel cast adrift without a compass.

Anger, anxiety and grief are common. None of these feelings is conducive to sustaining intimate relationships and rewarding sex. Once the adjustment has been made, a couple can move on with life. However, if this anxiety is carried on, this can be destructive not only to personal relationships but also to sex life. Anxiety can interfere with how the drugs work and the severity of symptoms. Tremor and dyskinesia are both increased by anxiety as are "off" periods. It can be difficult to determine cause and effect but the result is the same. Anxiety can infect the very people who care most about the person with Parkinson's and their anxiety feeds his/hers and vice-versa.

We would like to suggest some guidelines for a couple seeking help:

1. Often desire is still very much present, but there are physical difficulties and a referral to a sexual medicine clinic is appropriate. In the man, several changes take place with normal aging that can be made worse sooner by the presence of Parkinsonism. The size and firmness of the erect penis is reduced. The erection may take longer to form, but sometimes the ejaculation occurs too quickly–this is termed "premature ejaculation." This may cause the man to hurry on to intercourse while it is still possible. However, the brevity of any sexual touching before and the reduction in the time of intercourse itself may well leave the partner frustrated and unsatisfied. She may even feel used. In contrast, ejaculation can also take much longer, such that the erection fails through fatigue before it takes place at all.

   There are several methods available to enhance the male erection to allow intercourse. In the UBC clinic, the majority of couples choose self-injection of one of the nerve messengers involved in the erection process. Parkinsonism can impair small movements of the hands and so sometimes partners help with the injection. There are other ways to enhance erections medically, but one very important non-medical option is to capitalize on sexual and intimate touching that does not involve intercourse.

2. If the man wants a referral for erection difficulties, care must be taken to ensure that intervention will not result in one partner being restored to sexual health, in other words, able to get and keep an erection, while the other is secretly angry and distraught at the prospect of resumed sexual relations. A referral to a urologist without prior counseling for both partners can be disastrous (think of getting a new toy and being told you can not use it). The anxiety, guilt and resentment that can flood these situations need to be addressed. These experiences of anxiety and resentment actually make the physical sexual problem worse. Staff trained in sexual medicine can be very helpful in integrating the physical with the emotional. It is not easy for couples (even those married for many years) to talk freely about this, but human beings can communicate with words: this is what sets us apart. However, many of us are inhibited when it comes to discussion about what we like and want in our physical relationships. Saying "Please put your hand here," "That is rather uncomfortable," "I really like it when you do that," should be so simple with a partner we love and trust but inhibition often gets in the way.

3. A female partner or patient may well have passed through menopause. For some women this represents a period of new vitality and enthusiasm. However, physical changes due to lack of estrogen, may take place in the female genitalia that result in a thinning of the walls of the

vagina and the labia. Entry of the penis can be uncomfortable due to dryness and loss of elasticity, and urinary tract irritation can occur. The hood over the clitoris and the lips get thinner too and stimulation may begin to hurt rather than excite. Both vaginal and bladder infection is more common, making it very difficult for the woman to want to be sexual. Estrogen replacement can reverse all of these changes. Once weekly vaginal estrogen cream can be used if the woman or her doctor prefer to avoid giving estrogen to the rest of her body.

4. Fatigue and whether the drugs are working reliably are important factors for determining the quality of orgasm in both sexes. Patients of both sexes report that orgasms are weaker, more like a loosely wound ball of knitting wool than a coiled spring. Sometimes muscle rigidity is more intense after orgasm but tremor is better. Having an orgasm during intercourse for many women with or without Parkinsonism may be difficult. Women may need some added stimulation in order to achieve orgasm. This is where the ability to communicate your needs so that your partner understands is so important. If we can speak about these kinds of concerns, solutions can be found. For instance, the pleasuring she needs could take place after his ejaculation, or medical help to preserve the erection could be given. Parkinsonism is not usually associated directly with difficulties reaching orgasm.

5. A major problem arises when there is conflict between a couple about the frequency of sexual relationships. Most often, one wants more than the other, who may not want any at all. Frequently the male partner wishes to pursue sexual relations and is unable to because of erection problems. Anxiety, depression, the immobility associated with Parkinsonism and the drugs may contribute to this. Often the female partner does not care and is quite happy that sex has stopped. Sometimes there is a battle because one wants to, and can not but proceeds to try nevertheless, while the other lies there wishing that everything would stop.

In an attempt to see both sides of the picture we should understand that the symptoms of Parkinsonism result in a slow but relentless loss of autonomy with a commensurate increase in dependency. Thus, it is understandable that the male patient who has given up work, driving, and sports, etc., may wish to assert his authority and independence through his sexuality. The female partner needs to see his point of view and try to improve his self esteem by praising his successes outside the bedroom. Many of the patients we see are certain their sexual desire is increased by the dopaminergic drugs. This applies to both men and women. This can lead to sadness in the partner who wonders if "maybe it is only the drugs, it is not really making love." Realizing that it is likely that the drugs are, in fact, allowing the sexual feelings to become conscious and that without the drugs they stay hidden, can often be helpful.

6. Our need for a sexual relationship and how receptive we are to advances from another depend so much on external forces. In addition to inevitable stressors such as finances, family and work problems, for people with Parkinsonism, there is even more to contend with. The medications and their side effects, the illness, symptoms and fatigue, can all combine to interfere with normal responses on the part of both partners.

Fatigue plays a huge role in the disruption of sexual relations and intimacy in good health. In Parkinsonism, fatigue is due to the fact that everyday tasks are taking much longer and require more conscious effort; sleep can be disturbed, and the drugs tend to lower blood pressure which can make one feel tired. Both partners are possibly both sleep deprived if one of you needs help to go to the bathroom or to turn over in bed. It is similar to remembering what it was like with small babies in the house! It is necessary to be selfish and creative in choosing a time and place for sex, as the last thing at night is not the best time. Unplug the phone and enjoy some privacy when it seems right, at whatever time suits both partners.

If there are still children at home, spontaneity may be impossible. Try to schedule private dates at times when neither of you is exhausted. Few older children and teenagers are up before the sun and almost all go to bed later than their parents. Setting the alarm a bit earlier in the morning gives couples some uninterrupted private time together when both are rested.

7. Women make up the largest group of caregivers in America. When a woman provides care to a male mate there may be significant changes in the balance of the relationship. She may be assuming the responsibility for bill paying, taxes, insurance, etc., that impose on her time and can increase her anxiety. This may be a repetition of the care she gave her children and her parents and in-laws. These often intimate tasks may impinge on her ability to continually view her partner as sexually attractive and desirable. In addition in Parkinsonism, the change in body image, tremor, dyskinesia, lack of facial expression, skin texture, and smell (the drugs may cause a change in body odor for some) may make a person of either sex seem less attractive to their partner at the very time when their self esteem is crumbling and they need encouragement. These kind of changes can be difficult for both the patient and partner. In the Queen's Square study of 37 couples, one of whom had Parkinsonism, Brown et al., found that female partners had more difficulties with their sex lives than female patients (1990). The partner

in better health can feel guilty about seeming to impose his or her sexual needs on the other. Some people worry that it might be wrong for someone who is "ill" to be sexual. The media certainly does not help with its portrayal that sex is for the healthy young (and beautiful).

The adjustment within a relationship may vary enormously from a cessation of all sexual relations to maintaining essentially normal relations (for the relationship) with only minor changes. As long as both partners accept the situation, no intervention should be contemplated. The difficulty comes when one wants more than the other can give. There is much written about a woman's need to be held and stroked in a way that will not always lead to sex. Surely, there must be some men who like being held and caressed without the need to proceed further? So often within a partnership the refusal of sexual advances causes enormous hurt to the person being rebuffed. The reverse happens when the person wanting sex does not realize that the advances are assuming nightmarish proportions whether or not the sex act is completed. Women have used the words "rape" and "violated" to describe these persistent unwanted and incomplete attempts. The bedroom should not be a battleground. If no understanding or compromise can be reached, then separate bedrooms should be an option.

This paper has, thus far, assumed that sex takes place within a partnership. There are plenty of people with Parkinsonism who are single by choice, chance or through widowhood. They are straight and gay. They marry and divorce after diagnosis, conceive and bear children, change partners. They are totally normal in that regard. Particular difficulties arise for men and women living in nursing homes. Sadly, nursing staff can be very judgmental about the sexual needs of these residents. The fact is the facility is their home. Men and women may be used to masturbating regularly, for example. Masturbation is not an aberration and staff can respect the privacy of residents by knocking on doors and withdrawing discretely. Some men without partners and, to a lesser extent, some women may be used to paying for their sex. While it is unreasonable to allow paid sex in the facility, arrangements can be made for a resident to go to a pre-arranged appointment for it, if that is their wish. Conjugal visits with uninterrupted time can be allowed for men and women alike.

The sex drive may increase in a few men with late stage Parkinsonism in the presence of some memory loss and disinhibition. Some researchers feel that dopaminergic drugs contribute to this. This situation is difficult both in the home and in a facility. It disturbs everyone including the patient who experiences great agitation and frustration. A first step is to help the staff understand why the person is acting this way, and to discuss practical ways to reduce the negative consequences of the behavior. Following this, a trial of medication to reduce the effects of the male testosterone may allow the patient to remain living where he is with restored dignity when, without treatment, a psychiatric facility might be the only alternative. It may take considerable time and patience to ensure the patient understands that the medication is to relieve his agitation and frustration from having so much sexual drive and his shame from the consequences of it. The medications used do not take the drive away, but may reduce it.

In summary, that precious aspect of our lives that is often overlooked medically, namely our sexuality, may indeed be affected if one has Parkinsonism. The role changes, the losses, the change in appearance and non-sexual abilities, may alter sexual self-image and sexual attractiveness to the partner. These changes are real and negative feelings about them are legitimate. Talking about them is the beginning of their acceptance and allows moving on with continued but different kinds of physical intimacy. Physical changes may result from Parkinsonism disease, especially difficulties with erection, and these can be treated. Partner involvement in the treatment is vital. Incidental to Parkinsonism but very commonly the cause of sexual dysfunction, lack of estrogen after menopause, may add further problems or indeed may only come to light after the erections have been improved medically. These changes due to estrogen lack are all treatable. The decision to decline medical intervention if intercourse becomes impossible, but instead, to find more ways of intimate, physical sexual enjoyment without the act of intercourse, remains a very real and rewarding option. There is often a great sadness when all physical and sexual intimacy stops because that one component of our sexuality, namely, intercourse, becomes difficult or impossible. For most of us, the need to be physically cherished continues and this remains true even if we have Parkinsonism.

REFERENCES

Brown RG, Jahanschi M, Quinn N, Marsden CD. Sexual Function in Patients with Parkinson's Disease and Their Partners. J Neurol Neurosurg and Psych 1990;53:480-486.

Carlton L., Sex, Love and Chronic Illness. 1994. The National Parkinson Foundation Inc. (Miami).

Lipe H, Longstreth WT, Bird TD, Linde M. Sexual function in married men with Parkinson's disease compared to married men with arthritis. Neurology 1990;40:1347-1349.

Genetic Counseling
and Parkinson's Disease

Deborah de Leon

What exactly is genetic counseling? It is a process where the hereditary basis of a condition present in a family is explored. First, an accurate diagnosis of the condition is essential, and a thorough family history must be constructed. Sometimes medical and laboratory examinations of affected individuals and family members need to be conducted. What is known and not known about the genetic basis of the disorder is reviewed and education about inheritance patterns is provided. Concerns about implications to family members are addressed, and options for dealing with any identified risks are discussed, such as whether any specific genetic testing is available.

It is being learned that genes play an enormously important role in predisposition to diseases, especially the neurological disorders. Parkinson's disease (PD) may not be a single disorder. Parkinsonism can be thought of as a syndrome or a group of diseases, with many different causes, some which are genetic and others purely environmental. Research studies are now being conducted on PD and the role of genetics. Molecular genetic studies looking for a particular causative gene are being done at Columbia Presbyterian Medical Center and at other institutions. Once a gene or genes are found that cause or increase one's susceptibility to PD, many issues will be raised in families and genetic counseling will be one way to address them.

Genetic counseling is a fairly new field, and the National Society of Genetic Counselors is only twenty years old with about 1000 members worldwide. Genetic counselors usually have Master's level training in human

Deborah de Leon, MS, is Genetic Counselor, Center for Parkinson's Disease and Other Movement Disorders, Columbia Presbyterian Center, New York Presbyterian Hospital, New York.

[Haworth co-indexing entry note]: "Genetic Counseling and Parkinson's Disease." de Leon, Deborah. Co-published simultaneously in *Loss, Grief & Care* (The Haworth Press, Inc.) Vol. 8, No. 3/4, 2000, pp. 29-31; and: *Parkinson's Disease and Quality of Life* (ed: Côté et al.) The Haworth Press, Inc., 2000, pp. 29-31. Single or multiple copies of this article are available for a fee from The Haworth Document Delivery Service [1-800-342-9678, 9:00 a.m. - 5:00 p.m. (EST). E-mail address: getinfo@haworthpressinc.com].

genetics, with special training in counseling for genetic disorders. Genetic counselors often work together in teams with medical geneticists (physicians with specialty training in human genetic diseases). At Columbia, genetic counselors work with neurologists who specialize in movement disorders.

There are several different ways that genetic disorders can be passed on or inherited in families. Drawing and studying the family tree is one of the tools used to determine how a disease is inherited in a family. Some genetic disorders are inherited in an autosomal dominant fashion. This means that individuals with the disorder will appear in each generation, and that a gene is passed down from one generation directly to the next. A parent with a dominant genetic disease has a 50% chance to pass on that disease to each child. There are reports of some very large families with PD that look like they fit this pattern. It is not yet clear how much of PD is inherited in this fashion.

Another type of inheritance pattern is called autosomal recessive and this is where both parents are carrying a gene for the condition, but neither of them have the condition themselves. However, when the two genes come together in a child, the child can be affected, and there is a 25% chance for carrier parents to have an affected child. There could also be normal children and you can also have children who are carrying the gene. Some common examples of this are Tay-Sachs disease in Ashkenazi Jews, sickle-cell anemia in African Americans, and cystic fibrosis in caucasians. It is not yet known whether any PD is inherited in this fashion.

Another inheritance pattern is called X-linked recessive. In this pattern, only males are affected with the disorder, and females are the carriers of the gene for the disorder. Hemophilia is inherited in this fashion. A rare form of Parkinsonism is caused in this fashion, exclusive to Philippine males, and dystonia is also present in the disorder.

It is also possible to have a gene, like a dominant gene, that causes susceptibility to a disease, but other environmental factors need to be present, either some types of insults that one has been exposed to or some other unknown factors, for the disorder to actually be apparent. This is referred to as multifactorial inheritance, meaning many different factors have to be present—susceptibility genes and environmental factors. More research is needed to determine how PD is inherited, and how many different genetic types exist.

There are some concrete things that we can do now for our children and families, and our parents can do for us. One of them is recording the family history very carefully. When older generations in a family are gone that information may be lost and often there will be no other source in the family who knew anything about previous generations. Also consider becoming involved in research, especially if there are two or more living relatives in your family who have PD. Large families are important to study. Blood samples can also be banked for the purpose of storing genetic material for future use. If a genetic test becomes available in the future to diagnose a specific genetic type of PD, family members may need a sample of blood from deceased relatives to confirm the type of PD and to determine whether they carry the gene or not. There are commercial laboratories where blood can be banked for this purpose. Consider allowing an autopsy upon death to confirm the diagnosis of the type of PD, and also consider brain donation for research.

Sexuality and Parkinson's

Donna J. Dorros

Sexuality can be defined as a pattern of learned human conduct, including not only certain skills and behavior, but also feelings and attitudes people have about themselves as sexual beings. How we arrive at our own sexuality depends on how we were treated by our parents, our peers, and society's expectations by virtue of our being male or female. More than the act of copulating, it is the body signals, the eye contact, the caressing and fondling, as well as the caring of one individual for another. When this definition is combined with that of "disability," i.e., any condition that limits functioning to the fullest extent, one comes up with a number of misconceptions. The first is that the only proper sexual expression is intercourse, with both partners achieving orgasm at the same time. Another one is that sexuality and feelings of love are only for the young and the beautiful, particularly as portrayed by the mass media. Studies have debunked the notion that aging causes sexual desires to cease. A third misconception is that disabled people, such as Parkinsonians, are "noble sufferers" and do not indulge in pleasurable activities such as sex. It is important to remember that our sexuality is the birthright for each of us, not something that we have earned, nor something we have lost because of Parkinson's.

Despite the importance of our sexuality, it is a topic that most patients, caregivers and even doctors are reluctant to discuss. There seems to be an embarrassment or stigma attached to the subject which prevents individuals from being open and honest about their worries or fears. Parkinsonism can erode not only one's ability to move upon command, but also one's self-image and feelings of sexual attractiveness. In fact, some patients feel that they can no longer be interested in or capable of being sexually active. They may even look upon themselves as challenged, and therefore unable to have

Donna J. Dorros is a Parkinson widow, Gaithersburg, MD.

[Haworth co-indexing entry note]: "Sexuality and Parkinson's." Dorros, Donna J. Co-published simultaneously in *Loss, Grief & Care* (The Haworth Press, Inc.) Vol. 8, No. 3/4, 2000, pp. 33-35; and: *Parkinson's Disease and Quality of Life* (ed: Côté et al.) The Haworth Press, Inc., 2000, pp. 33-35. Single or multiple copies of this article are available for a fee from The Haworth Document Delivery Service [1-800-342-9678, 9:00 a.m. - 5:00 p.m. (EST). E-mail address: getinfo@haworthpressinc.com].

anything to do with sex. However, whether or not they have Parkinson's, they still have sexual desires. Whether they can *perform* or not, the desire is still there. Patients may have some form of sexual dysfunction brought on by the disease process or the medication or simply lack of sexual confidence. For male patients, such dysfunction may result in premature ejaculation or inability to achieve or maintain a penile erection. Many times these conditions are amenable to medical treatment.

For caregivers there may be problems, as well. They may not understand their partner's sexual needs, or they may be worn down with work and/or care giving. Also, there may be stress, frustration, or tension in the family. In long term relationships, the sex act over time may have become mechanical or just a habit that has very little meaning.

In order to overcome these and other attitudes which may be prevalent in Parkinson patients and their spouses, it is important to learn how to communicate. You may have to begin by building confidence in each other about your sexual desires. Learn how to break down your respective hang-ups and to express these individual needs. Showing concern and interest in one another can make each partner feel loved and wanted. Perhaps you start out by something as simple as holding hands. You should not try to rush it. Good communication takes time. Being kind to one another, touching, and caressing, can break down barriers and lead to further sexual expression. If you find it impossible to achieve the kind of communication you are seeking on your own, it might be worth it to explore professional counseling.

The simple act of touching can make a Parkinsonian feel less handicapped and more secure. When Sid became immobile, I would usually give him a hug. Often, he could then initiate movement. We believed in and practiced hugging several times a day, in addition to other ways of showing that we cared for and had sexual feelings for one another. At the times when sexual intercourse is not possible, you need not deprive yourself or your partner of sexual pleasure. The act of cuddling, kissing, or tender stroking between you and your mate can be very satisfying and may even lead to intercourse. If not, you have at least given one another a sense of closeness and caring. A fulfilling, intimate relationship with another human being is one of give and take. In order for it to be gratifying for both of you, neither should do all the giving or all the taking because each person has their own needs.

As in all aspects of coping with a chronic illness, there is a delicate balancing act of adequate rest, exercise, diet, medication, positive emotions, controlling of stress, and most important of all–giving and accepting love. As the Parkinsonian learns to accommodate to his or her limitations, so must the care partner. Careful timing and flexibility become very important. This may take some attitude adjustment and new ways of doing things for both of you. It can be difficult to adjust to the changes which occur in a previously healthy spouse after a chronic illness such as Parkinson's is diagnosed. Concern over these changes should be discussed openly between both parties, especially as they relate to sexuality. If not, they can escalate to serious proportions.

The Parkinsonian should be functioning well before attempting sexual activity. This is usually early in the day and within thirty minutes after taking medication. The care partner should feel comfortable about adapting to his or her desires regardless of the time of day. Try making a "date" with one another. That will give each of you time to plan ahead and to develop amorous feelings.

Do not overlook the importance of careful grooming and hygiene to enhance the experience. It may help set the mood by playing romantic music, wearing provocative apparel and using sensual fragrances. Try being inventive and creative. What this may mean depends on the people involved.

When my husband, Sid, and I started seeing one another in a romantic relationship, we were both past fifty years of age, and he was already in an advanced stage of Parkinsonism. To some that would have been the ultimate put off, but if you love, admire, and respect one another you can realize sexual fulfillment despite the obvious difficulties. What becomes important is not the fact that one of you has a chronic neurological illness, but that you love one another and find happiness being together. A solid basis for a lasting relationship is friendship and respect. We had that for a number of years so when we found that our feelings for one another were growing deeper, it was not too difficult to overcome the inevitable problems of Parkinson's and the side effects of the medications. In a way, it was an advantage to begin a relationship with an awareness of these problems instead of having them thrust upon you at a later time. We both felt that the joy of discovering love and sexual pleasure despite Parkinson's disease and middle age was a great gift. We found that love can actually be better and more satisfying as you grow older, despite the myths.

We savored our sexual relationship right up to the time of Sid's death even though we, too, experienced occasional problems brought on by the inexorable progression of thirty years with Parkinson's. Sid's last request from me was a hug–which, of course, he got!

Use of Animals in Scientific Research, Education and Testing

Ralph B. Dell

The use of animals in scientific research, education and testing requires knowing and complying with the rules and regulations that pertain to the use of animals in research and understanding the ethics of the use of animals. The reason that animals are used is that whole animals are complex and integrated biological systems and, while much can be learned from isolated systems, ultimately research has to be done in the whole animal. Such research is performed to understand how many, independent systems are integrated into the whole organism. And, in fact, much of the progress that we've made in both basic science and in medical research has required the use of whole animals. While animals must be used in research, it is recognized that scientists have a moral and ethical responsibility to use animals humanely and responsibly.

This article will summarize the use of animals in biomedical research. The references at the end of this article give more detail on many aspects of research that uses animals. First, the rules and regulations will be discussed briefly. Then the role of the committee that oversees the rules and regulations at an institution will be considered along with some of the ethical issues and principles that are involved in the use of animals. Finally, I'll make a couple of observations relating to the use of animals in Parkinson's disease research based upon our experience at Columbia. This article should serve as an introduction to the topic.

Two federal agencies have rules and administer laws that affect the use of

Ralph B. Dell, MD, is Professor of Pediatrics, College of Physicians and Surgeons, Institutional Animal Care and Use Committee, Health Sciences Division, Columbia University, New York, NY 10032.

[Haworth co-indexing entry note]: "Use of Animals in Scientific Research, Education and Testing." Dell, Ralph B. Co-published simultaneously in Loss, Grief & Care (The Haworth Press, Inc.) Vol. 8, No. 3/4, 2000, pp. 37-40; and: Parkinson's Disease and Quality of Life (ed: Côté et al.) The Haworth Press, Inc., 2000, pp. 37-40. Single or multiple copies of this article are available for a fee from The Haworth Document Delivery Service [1-800-342-9678, 9:00 a.m. - 5:00 p.m. (EST). E-mail address: getinfo@haworth.pressinccom].

animals in research: the United States Department of Agriculture and the Public Health Service. In New York State a third agency also regulates the use of animals in research, the New York State Department of Health. The United States Department of Agriculture's regulations apply to all warm blooded animals excluding rats, mice and birds. These regulations are enforced by inspectors who perform unannounced inspections of all research facilities annually. The Public Health Service regulations cover all vertebrate animals. Enforcement depends upon an assurance from the institution that describes how the institution will comply with all regulations. Site visits are performed for cause, that is, if there have been complaints about the care and use of laboratory animals at an institution, the Public Health Service will investigate. A New York State Department of Health inspector conducts yearly unannounced inspections of all registered animal facilities in the State. New York's regulations cover all vertebrates.

The Public Health Service regulations and United States Department of Agriculture regulations have many features in common. For example, both call for a committee to oversee the use of animals at an institution. The committee is composed of at least one veterinarian, one scientist, one non-scientist, and a member who is unaffiliated with the institution in any way. At this institution we have eighteen members on the committee with three veterinarians, eleven biomedical research scientists, three non-scientists and one unaffiliated member. The duties of this committee are to inspect every six months the facilities where animals are housed and to review all institutional programs for caring for animals. These programs include such items as veterinary care, frequency of cage cleaning, methods for safely handling hazardous agents, and the like. The committee is charged with reviewing any concerns that anyone has with the care of animals. Finally, the committee also reviews all animal use protocols. These are documents written by scientists describing in detail how the animal is to be used in the proposed research. Thus, there are extensive federal and state laws and regulations that govern the use of animals in research that must be adhered to by all people who use animals in research, education and testing.

Next, some of the ethical issues surrounding the use of animals in scientific research will be considered. Most people who have studied this issue ultimately use a utilitarian or a risk benefit analytical approach to study this problem. The benefit to people is that research using animals has led to improvements in the health of both humans and animals due to the advancement of science, both basic and applied. It is important to realize that people are living longer and healthier lives than they were 50 years ago. Most of the improvements in the health of people as well as advances in veterinary medicine have depended upon the use of animals in research. Nearly 3/4 of all of the Nobel prizes that have been given in this century in Medicine and

Physiology have been given for research that used animals for some part of the prize winning research. The potential benefit of using animals in research is high. This is not to say that all research is of prize winning quality but that, overall, tremendous progress is being made. Secondly, most people who think about these issues accept the idea of kinship and hierarchy. Man has the right, if not obligation, to consider the human species first over all other animals. Tempering this hierarchical view of the animal kingdom is the realization that man has the moral responsibility to use animals as humanely and responsibly as possible. In summary, these are the conclusions reached by most people who have studied this issue. There is obviously another view of the ethics of using animals in research which uses the ideas of rights. People holding this view of the use of animals by mankind deny that there is a hierarchy. They hold that all animals have the capacity to experience pain and distress, that is, have the capacity to suffer. They further hold that all animals have a right not to suffer and not to experience pain and distress and therefore the people who use this analytical approach come to the conclusion that mankind does not have the right to use animals in life saving research.

Ethical principles for the use of animals in research have been developed by the United States Government. Entitled the United States Government Principles for the Care and Use of Laboratory Animals in Medical Research, these principles state that all procedures that use animals must be designed so that they are relevant to the improvement of health, the advancement of knowledge, or the good of society. Further, the scientist must use an appropriate model and must consider alternatives to the use of animals. Alternatives to the use of animals include not only replacement by non-animal methods but also use of the lowest species possible and use of experimental design that avoid or minimize pain and distress. Appropriate sedation, analgesia and anesthesia must be used when the proposed procedure is invasive. It is the responsibility of the investigator to euthanize all animals that are suffering severe or chronic pain. The animal care committee must assess protocols for the use of animals using these principles.

At Columbia Presbyterian Medical Center we have had considerable experience with the use of animals in Parkinson's disease research. Early in these experiments the animals were quite ill and difficult to care for, requiring extraordinary measures to maintain and support the animals. This early experience led to a re-evaluation of the research methodology to determine if it would be possible to explore efficacy of the new therapeutic modalities with a less severe form of Parkinson's disease. A less invasive method for doing the research has been developed. Now animals are independent and able to care for themselves but exhibit the signs and symptoms of Parkinson's disease in sufficient strength so that one can evaluate the various forms of the new therapies that are being investigated. This is a good example of the interaction that exists between the scientist, the animal care committee, and the veterinarians involved in the care of the animals so that, over a period of time, methods have been devised that are less traumatic and less invasive for the animal.

In summary, this is a brief overview of the federal and state rules and regulations that govern the use of animals in research, some of the ethical issues involved in the use of animals in medical research, and our experiences in using animals in Parkinson's Disease research.

REFERENCES

Biosafety in Microbiological and Biomedical Laboratories. Centers for Disease Control, Fall 1992.

Education and Training in the Care and Use of Laboratory Animals. National Research Council, 1991.

Fox, J.G., Cohen, B.J., Loew, F.M., Laboratory Animal Medicine. Academic Press, Inc., 1984.

Guide for the Care and Use of Agricultural Animals in Agricultural Research and Teaching (Agri-Guide). American Dairy Science Association, 1989.

Guide for the Care and Use of Laboratory Animals. National Institutes of Health, 1985-6.

Institutional Animal Care and Use Committee Guidebook. U.S. Department of Health and Human Services, Public Health Service, National Institutes of Health Publ. No. 92-3415.

Institutional Administrator's Guide for Animal Care and Use. National Institutes of Health, 1988.

Principles and Guidelines for Use of Animals in Precollege Education. Institute of Laboratory Animal Resources, 1989.

Public Health Service Policy on Humane Care and Use of Laboratory Animals. National Institutes of Health, 1986.

Report of the AVMA Panel on Euthanasia. American Veterinary Medical Association, 1986.

The Biomedical Investigators Handbook for Researchers Using Animal Models. Foundation for Biomedical Research. Washington, DC 1987.

Genetic Factors
in Parkinson's Disease

Roger C. Duvoisin

Most of us know the parents or grandparents we come from. But we go back and back, forever; we go back all of us to the very beginning; in our blood and bone and brain we carry the memories of thousands of beings. . . .

V. S. Naipaul

INTRODUCTION

When I have addressed audiences throughout the U.S. and Canada the past several years, I have found that typically about a third of the audience was aware of other family members who also had Parkinson's disease (PD). The proportion grows closer to one half among those who had extensive knowledge of their family tree and know about all four grandparents, both parents, all uncles and aunts as well as all siblings. Even that proportion underestimates the true prevalence of Parkinson's disease among their relatives for, due to the late average age of symptom onset many die of natural causes before developing sufficient symptoms to be diagnosed. Moreover, some relatives will experience only one or two symptoms, tremor only or trouble walking for example, which is ascribed to something else such as essential

Roger C. Duvoisin was Willliam Dow Lovett Professor of Neurology and Chairman, Department of Neurology, University of Medicine and Dentistry of New Jersey, New Jersey's University of Health Sciences, Robert Wood Johnson Medical School, New Brunswick, NJ when this article was written.

[Haworth co-indexing entry note]: "Genetic Factors in Parkinson's Disease." Duvoisin, Roger C. Co-published simultaneously in *Loss, Grief & Care* (The Haworth Press, Inc.) Vol. 8, No. 3/4, 2000, pp. 41-53; and: *Parkinson's Disease and Quality of Life* (ed: Côté et al.) The Haworth Press, Inc., 2000, pp. 41-53. Single or multiple copies of this article are available for a fee from The Haworth Document Delivery Service [1-800-342-9678, 9:00 a.m. - 5:00 p.m. (EST). E-mail address: getinfo@haworthpressinc.com].

tremor or arthritis or old age. Some people are probably aware of several cases in their family tree going back three or four generations in a pattern consistent with hereditary transmission. Considering the late age of onset of PD on average, this is remarkable evidence of familial aggregation. It is somewhat embarrassing that this evidence has been better recognized by patients and their families than by their physicians.

The fact that PD can occur in several members of a family over two or more generations has been known for well over a century and has long suggested an important role for heredity in the cause of the disease. Recent reports of well documented multicase families in which true PD has occurred in a clearly hereditary pattern in successive generations have made it clear that PD can occur on a genetic basis. There has been a growing awareness that many cases of PD are familial. Studies of familial PD have now provided compelling evidence that PD is a genetic disorder. To some this news may be disturbing because of the fear that a genetic cause will present enormous scientific and ethical difficulties. Moreover, the idea that the cause lies within ourselves in our genes strikes at our very sense of being. It also raises a host of new and troubling questions. Will other family members and in particular the children someday be subject to the same illness? Could we diagnose the presence of the gene before there are any symptoms? If so, would we really want to?

The renewed interest in the genetics of PD should be seen in a more positive light because it brings forward the possibility of finally clarifying the cause and fundamental mechanism of the disease. Given the multicase PD families and the remarkable power of modern DNA molecular analysis it is virtually certain a responsible gene mutation will be found. It is merely a matter of time and effort. Here then lies the quickest and surest road to means of prevention and cure. Geneticists have already begun to examine multiple-case families seeking to clarify the patterns of inheritance and collecting blood samples from which the DNA can be isolated for molecular analysis in search of a "Parkinson gene." At the time of writing, the search is well underway and it is likely that the location of such a gene on a particular chromosome may soon be found!

THE HISTORIC STUDY OF MJÖNES

The first serious systematic genetic study of PD was carried out nearly a half-century ago by a young psychiatrist, Dr. Henry Mjönes (1949) at the University of Lund in Sweden. He was working for an advanced doctoral degree in medicine under the guidance of Professor Sjögren, a noted pioneer of medical genetics. Dr. Mjönes identified 194 patients with PD and studied their families for the presence of secondary cases. He found that 43% of the patients had one or more affected relatives. In all, there were 162 secondary cases. He also found nine families in which PD was known to have occurred in successive generations. Mjönes concluded that PD was a genetic disorder with considerable variation in symptoms and age of onset. His report, however, was largely ignored and it was some years before further studies were carried out.

Subsequent studies designed to asses how often PD was familial were inconclusive; several found some evidence of a familial pattern but the number of cases were too small, the families were usually not examined by the investigators and there was confusion regarding the interpretation of relatives affected with minimal or atypical symptoms. The attempt to resolve the question of the role of heredity in PD with studies of identical twins failed to find a high rate of concordance for PD but as Johnson et al. pointed out (1990) the results were inconclusive, chiefly due to the difficulty of finding a sufficient number of twins and uncertainty in the interpretation of atypical features. More recent studies of twins with PET scanning of co-twins who were either apparently unaffected or had too few symptoms to permit the diagnosis have indicated that the concordance rate is much higher than the earlier studies had indicated (Burn, Mark, Playford et al., 1992).

MULTICASE FAMILIES

Mjönes' Families

The major impetus for renewed study of the genetics of PD has been the rediscovery in the past decade of families in which PD clearly occurs in a hereditary pattern for these have shown that PD can be genetically determined. In his historic study, Mjönes had found a number of families in which PD had appeared in successive generations. An example of one of these multiply affected families is described here. The proband–the member of the family first identified by Mjönes–is marked by the arrow. This woman had developed typical PD symptoms in the 1940's at age 61. Her brother developed PD symptoms at age 62. Her father had had only a tremor for many years and lived to age 85. One of her father's sisters also had PD. Her son had the onset of PD at age 27. He had no tremor. Her paternal grandfather was reported by the family to also have had PD. He was born in 1823 and lived to age 83. The proband closely resembled her grandfather in her symptoms.

This family illustrates some of the problems which have confounded efforts to assess the role of genetic factors in PD. Some affected family members fail to develop all the symptoms. Indeed, they may have only one or two even after many years. The father had only one symptom–tremor–and if he were not part of the family he might be dismissed as a case of essential tremor. In contrast, the son had no tremor and had an early age of onset in his twenties. Considered independently of the family he would be apt to be diagnosed with some condition other than PD. Mjönes accepted such atypically or minimally affected family members as secondary cases of PD. Unfortunately, he did not have post-mortem confirmation of the diagnosis of PD in such cases or other means of confirming the diagnosis. Although post-mortem studies were done in some of the patients he studied, these were of little help because the structural changes in the nervous system characteristic of PD were not then understood.

The Spellman-Muenter Pedigree

The first multicase family recorded in the medical literature in which post-mortem studies confirmed that the family disease was in fact PD was a large family from the midwest. A brief medical report of this family was published by Dr. George Spellman of Sioux City Iowa (1962). At that time nine members of the family were known to have been affected. The next generation of the family was encountered by Dr. Manfred Muenter of the Mayo Clinic in Rochester, Minnesota (Muenter et al., 1986). By that time, a total of 15 members of the family had been affected in 4 successive generations. Dr. Muenter and recently, Dr. Demetrios Maraganore, also of the Mayo Clinic, have continued to study the family. Additional members have since become affected. Initially, because of an unusually early age of onset and rather severe symptoms affected members, this family was thought to have some condition other than PD but post-mortem examinations in several deceased members have shown changes typical of PD. Family members studied more recently have had more typical symptoms. Some are minimally affected and have only isolated tremor (Maraganore and Muenter, personal communication, 1995).

The Contursi Pedigree

The largest known pedigree of familial Parkinsonism has been studied by my associate, Dr. Lawrence Golbe, in collaboration with Prof. Giuseppe Di'Iorio of the University of Naples, Italy (Golbe et al., 1990, 1993). We were aware in 1995 of 61 affected members of the last four generations. All shared a common ancestor 11 generations back who lived in the village of Contursi in southern Italy in the 18th century. Approximately half of the known affected members of the family live in the U.S. and are descendants of two members of the family who immigrated circa 1900; the remainder live in Italy. The large size of this family makes possible a detailed analysis of the pattern of inheritance, variations in the age of onset and clinical manifestations. Several important points have emerged thus far.

First, as was noted in the family described by Mjönes and in the Spellman-Muenter pedigree, there is a large variation in the age of symptom onset but there is also a trend to an earlier age of onset in successive generations, a phenomenon known as "anticipation." This may be of some importance because anticipation has recently been associated with a particular kind of DNA mutation. There is also a large variation in the symptoms. For example, some affected have no tremor while others have typical rest tremor. Some respond well to levodopa therapy but others do not. The risk of developing PD is equal in men and women in this pedigree.

Other Families

Small families were reported in medical journals from Spain (Gimenez-Roldan, 1986) and Japan (Inose, 1988). More recently. Dr. Cheryl Waters (1994) of the University of Southern California reported a 4-generation family and Dr. Zbignew Wszolek of the University of Nebraska and his colleagues (1993, 1995) have reported four families with mutiple cases of PD collected from the midwest. Dr. Golbe and others (1994) also reported a family from Pennsylvania. Two children in the last generation of that family developed spasms in the feet which are probably the initial symptoms of PD. Post-mortem confirmation of the diagnosis of PD was available in all of these families.

A listing of the ten families thus far reported in the literature with post-mortem confirmation is shown in Table 1. Additional families have also been reported without post-mortem confirmation but the clinical information available suggests that they do represent true PD. Many more have been described at various medical meetings but full reports have not yet been published. All these families appear to share the same pattern of autosomal dominant inheritance noted in the larger families or pedigrees described above.

RECENT GENETIC STUDIES OF FAMILIAL PD

Dr. Maraganore (1991) working with Drs. Haarding and Marsden studied the families of 23 patients with positive family histories culled from a neurological clinic in London. These familial cases represented 16% of the PD patients seen at that clinic. Dr. Maraganore personally examined the reportedly affected relatives and found evidence of hereditary transmission of the disorder. He also compared the familial with sporadic cases drawn from the same clinic and found no differences in their signs or symptoms.

TABLE 1. Data from published reports of multiple-case families of Parkinson's disease confirmed by post-mortem examination. The numbers have increased in some of these families as additional members have become affected in the years since the last report was published. For example, 22 members of the Spellman-Muenter pedigree and 61 members of the Contursi pedigree are now known to have been affected.

Authors	# Affected	M	F
Spellman, Muenter et al. (1986)	15	9	6
Gimenez-Roldan et al. (1986)	4	1	3
Inose et al. (1988)	4	0	4
Golbe et al. (1990, 1993)	44	26	18
Wszolek et al. (1993) Family A	7	4	3
Family B	7	6	1
Family C	11	8	3
Family D (1995)	18	6	12
Golbe et al. (1994) "K" Family	9	6	3
Waters & Miller (1994)	9	4	5
Mizutami et al.	3	2	1
Totals	128	70	58

Prevalence of Familial PD

Recently my colleague, Alice Lazzarini, an experienced genetic counselor, collected family history data on all my personal patients who were seen during the calendar year 1991–a total of 211 patients with clinically typical PD to assess the prevalence of familial PD (Lazzarini et al., 1994). Then I and my colleagues, Drs. Lawrence Golbe, Margery Mark, Jacob Sage and Thomas Zimmerman, examined as many of the reportedly affected living relatives as possible. This required three years and extensive travel throughout the U.S. We found that 48 or 22% of my patients had one or more relatives with definite PD. However, full information on all 1st and 2nd degree relatives could be obtained for only 40 patients! In this subset of patients with more complete pedigree information the proportion who had one or more definitely affected relatives rose to 40%. If we add the "probably" affected relatives, the proportion rises to 53%. Now, a year after the publication of the report of that study, the "probably" affected relatives have become "definitely" affected and several additional relatives have become affected so that our numbers underestimate the true prevalence of PD among these patients' families. We also could find no differences between the familial and the sporadic cases. We believe that many of the latter would become familial if more data were available on their families.

Genetic Analysis

In the same study, Lazzarini and Dr. Richard Myers of Boston University carried out a detailed statistical analysis of a total of 80 multicase families collected from our clinic. Two important findings emerged. First, a lifetable analysis showed that the cumulative lifetime risk of developing PD among the relatives of our patients was greater than 40%. Second, ancestral secondary cases were found only on one side of the family in nearly all (97%) of the families. These findings confirmed the historic findings of Mjönes and of Maraganore et al. cited above. Overall, these three studies together constitute persuasive evidence that (a) genetic factors are important in PD, (b) familial PD accounts for a substantial proportion of patients with clinically diagnosed PD and finally, and (c) familial PD is inherited as an autosomal dominant due to inheritance of a DNA mutation at a single major locus.

Autosomal Dominant Inheritance

To explain what "autosomal dominant" means it is necessary to briefly review some elements of genetics. In the nucleus of every cell in human beings are 23 pairs of chromosomes. They are called chromosomes, meaning "colored bodies," because they take the color of certain chemical stains which render them visible when viewed under a microscope. They exist in pairs, one received from each parent. Two of the chromosomes, named "X" and "Y," are the sex chromosomes. The remaining 22 pairs are called "autosomes." Males have a Y chromosome inherited from their fathers and an X inherited from their mothers. Females have two X chromosomes, one inherited from each parent. We can infer that the gene for PD cannot be on either of the sex chromosomes since the disease affects men and women with equal frequency. Hence, PD is an "autosomal" disorder.

The term "dominant" indicates that a single copy of the disease gene is sufficient to cause the disease. From this fact it is clear that on average, one half the offspring of an affected parent are at risk of developing the condition in question. In contrast, in "recessive" disorders such as cystic fibrosis, individuals carrying a single copy of the disease gene inherited from one parent plus a normal copy inherited from the other parent do not develop symptoms. They are carriers because they can transmit the gene to their progeny. Only those individuals who receive two copies of the disease gene will develop the disease. That means they must receive one copy from each parent and that both parents must be carriers. On average, only one in four children of parents both of whom are carriers will be at risk of developing the condition in question. In general, recessive disorders are relatively rare, while dominant disorders are more common.

We can infer from the genetic analyses of PD families discussed above that each offspring of an affected parent has a 50% chance of carrying the disease gene. However that does not mean that half the offspring will actually develop the disease. This is because "penetrance" is incomplete. Due to the late age of onset of PD, only some of those who inherit the disease gene are likely to develop symptoms within a normal lifetime. Since we have observed PD first developing as late as age 101, we can conclude that penetrance will remain incomplete even at age 100!

Genetic Counseling

While we do not have enough data yet to precisely calculate penetrance and fully account for the variability, we may roughly estimate that the risk of a relative developing symptoms of PD is more than the 2.5% risk of the population as a whole but something less than 50%. From the observation that the median age of onset in a general population is about age 75, we can roughly estimate that the risk cannot be more than 25%. It is probably substantially less than that. In general, "dominant" disorders tend to be quite variable in the nature and severity of their symptoms and this has been the case in the multicase families we have studied. Thus, some of the offspring will develop mild symptoms, as in the formes frustes we described above, which may not justify the clinical diagnosis of PD. Taking all these considerations into account, the actual lifetime risk to each offspring of developing overt PD may be estimated at only 10% to perhaps 15%.

Because PD is not uncommon, one would expect rare cases to have both parents affected. We have seen a small number of patients who had affected relatives on both sides. It seems likely that at least some of these patients may have inherited two copies of the Parkinson gene, one from each parent. Yet their disease did not seem different from that in other patients. This is not surprising since we know that in other dominantly inherited conditions having two copies of the disease gene does not seem to make any difference.

Taking all these facts and observations into account one can conclude that the risks to an offspring, considering all the other diseases and accidents that can happen over the course of a lifetime, should not be a cause of major concern. Nor would I recommend that unaffected relatives or offspring of a patient seek examination in the hope of finding out if they are at risk of being affected at some unknown time in the future. Our opinion on this would doubtless be different if we had a reliable and accurate diagnostic test and there were means of preventing or delaying the appearance of Parkinsonism.

THE SEARCH FOR THE PARKINSON GENE

Candidate Genes

The search for a gene mutation responsible for PD has already begun. Since there are an estimated 100,000 genes in the human genome, this is no small task. Thus, initial studies have focused on particular genes suggested by various theoretical considerations. We consider these "candidate" genes. For example, following up on the suggestion that a defect in the enzyme tyrosine hydroxylase, which regulates the conversion of tyrosine to L-Dopa, might be a cause, the gene for this enzyme has been studied by investigators in the U.S., in Germany and in Japan1 (Tanaka et al., 1990, Borde-Neuve et al., 1994, Gasser et al., 1994). A number of variations in the gene are known to occur among normal individuals. The investigators thus searched for an association between a DNA variation and the occurrence of PD. The results have been negative and this gene has been essentially excluded as a possible site of a mutation which could cause PD.

The gene for the enzyme monoamine oxidase (MAO) has also been studied because the toxic effect of MPTP is dependent on its conversion by MAO to the toxin MPP+. If an MPTP-like substance were responsible for PD, then perhaps a variation in MAO might be found to play a role in predisposing one to the effects of such a substance. Again, a number of investigators have examined the variations in this gene but have failed to find one which is more common in PD patients than in others (Kurth et al., 1993, Hotamisligil, 1994). The gene coding for the liver enzyme debrisoquin hydroxylase has also been examined with the thought that variations in the ability of the liver to detoxify toxic substances might be correlated with PD. Again, no connection with PD has been found (Kurth and Kurth, 1993, Bordet et al., 1994).

A number of other candidate genes have been studied for possible associations with PD (Gasser et al., 1994). I will not review them here but simply note that all appear to have been excluded as possible sites of a Parkinson gene mutation. These results leave us with no useful clues as to the possible location of the gene mutation responsible for PD. Thus geneticists have begun a systematic search of the entire human genome to map the Parkinson gene. This is a tedious task which will require considerable effort and some time to complete. It has been likened to searching for a needle in a haystack. However, it is possible, with presently available techniques, to scan the entire genome and investigators in a number of genetic research laboratories have already begun to do this. Some have joined in an international collaboration to share the burden and pool their expertise. Thus far, they have covered about half the genome in their search but have not yet found linkage of a DNA variation with PD. One cannot predict when it will be found. The good news at this point in time is that the search is underway and making progress. We have the means and the scientific tools to accomplish the job.

A Triplet Repeat Disorder?

A shortcut was suggested by the observation of anticipation in some Parkinson families. Anticipation has been associated in a number of hereditary nervous system disorders with a particular type of DNA variation. To understand this variation one must recall that the genetic code consists of four coding molecules represented in the shorthand of molecular genetics by the letters C,A, G and T. Throughout the genome there are sequences in which three of these molecules form long repeating sequences, for example, CAGCAGCAGCAG. . . . .and so on for 30 to 40 or more repeats. These are known as triplet repeat sequences. Enlargements of specific triplet repeat sequences have been found to underlie Huntington's disease, Myotonic dystrophy and a number of other adult onset chronic neurologic disorders (Ross et al., 1993). Anticipation has been noted in all these conditions. Thus, the possibility arises that PD might also be associated with a triplet repeat sequence.

Accordingly, one group of collaborators has begun searching for a triplet sequence enlargement. So far, they have looked for a CAG triplet enlargement but found none (Carrero-Valenzuela et al., 1995). That leaves the possibility of other triplet sequences such as a GGC sequence, and further studies are underway following this clue.

One can only speculate at present as to where the Parkinson gene mutation will eventually be found. Experience with other conditions suggests that it will prove to be a previously unknown gene. Presumably, it will code for a protein which is presently unknown. I have elsewhere suggested that the protein might be named "parkinsin" (Duvoisin, 1994). Once the gene is found and the protein identified, its function will be studied to determine how it may cause PD and to search for possible means of therapeutic intervention.

Transmission of the abnormal gene to experimental animals to form "transgenic" animal models of PD will probably be used to accelerate the study of the mechanism of the disease. For the first time, a true animal model of the disease would become possible. A transgenic Parkinson mouse could then be used to test methods of treatment. These might include methods of blocking, enhancing or modulating in some way the action of the abnormal protein "parkinsin." Or the gene itself could be the target of therapeutic attack. The idea that a human disease might be corrected at the genetic level has become an "established driving force in medicine" (Friedman, 1994). The technology, using viruses as vectors to carry to the diseased cells a desired segment of DNA, is still in its infancy but we may expect that it will grow rapidly in the years ahead.

CONCLUSION

In conclusion, there is now compelling evidence that PD is a genetic disorder. Families with multiple cases of PD are now well documented. Modern techniques of molecular analysis of DNA make it possible to map the location of the responsible gene mutation on the human genome in these families. The effort to map the gene is now underway and it appears probable that a gene locus will soon be found. Once the gene is identified and its function clarified, it will then be possible to clarify the mechanism of the disease process. Our understanding of PD will be profoundly changed and entirely new methods of treatment, prevention and even a cure will become possible.

REFERENCES

Barbeau A, Roy M (1984). Familial subsets in idiopathic in Parkinson's disease. Can J Neurosci;11:144-150.

Bordet R, Broly F, Destee A, Libersa C (1994). Genetic polymorphis, of cytochrome P450 2D6 in idiopathic Parkinson disease and diffuse Lewy body disease.Clin Neuropharmacol;17:484-488.

Burn DJ, Mark HM, Playford ED et al. Parkinson's disease twins studied with 18F-dopa and positron emission tomography. Neurology 1992;42:1894-1900.

Carrero-Valenzuela R, Lindblad K, Payami H, Johnson WG, Schalling M, Stenroos BA, Shattuc S, Nutt J, Brice A, Litt M (1995). No evidence for association of familial Parkinson disease with CAG repeat expansion. Neurology: in press.

Duvoisin RC (1994). Research on the genetics of Parkinson's disease: will it lead to the cause and a cure? In MB Stern, ed.: *Beyond the Decade of the Brain.* Wells Medical Ltd, Royal Tunbridge Wells, pp. 95-108.

Friedman T (1994). Gene therapy for neurological disorders. Trends Genet;10:210-213.

Gasser T, Wszolek ZK, Trofatter J., et al. (1994). Genetic linkage studies in autosomal dominant Parkinsonism: evaluation of seven candidate genes. Ann Neurol;36:368-372.

Giminez-Roldan S, Mateo D, Escalona-Zapata J (1986). Familial Alzheimer's disease presenting as levodopa-responsive parknsonism. Adv Neurol; 45:431-436.

Golbe LI, Di Iorio G, Bonavita V, Miller DC, Duvoisin RC (1990). A large kindred with autosomal dominant Parkinson's disease. Ann Neurol; 27: 276-282.

Golbe LI, Di Iorio G, Lazzarini AM, Bonavita V, Duvoisin RC (1993). A large kindred with Parkinson's disease (PD): onset age, segregation ratios and anticipation. [abstract, poster P3] Mov Disord; 8:406.

Golbe LI, Lazzarini AM, Schwarz KO et al. (1993). Autosomal dominant Parkinsonism with benign course and typical Lewy body pathology. Neurology 1993;43:2222-2227.

Hotamisligil GS, Girmen AS, Fink JS et al. (1994). Hereditary variations in monamine oxidase as a risk factor for Parkinson's disease. Mov Disord;9:305-310.

Inose T, Miyakawa M, Miyakawa K, Mizushima S, Oyanagi S, Ando S. (1988) Clinical and neuropatholoical study of juveile Parkinsonism. Jap J Psych & Neurol; 42: 265-276.

Johnson WG, Hodge SE, Duvoisin RC (1990). Twin studies and the genetics of Parkinson's disease. Mov Disord 5:187-194

Kurth JH, Kurth MC, Podusloi SE et al. (1993). Association of a monoamine oxidase B allele with Parkinson's disease. Ann Neurol; 33:368-372.

Kurth MC, Kurth JH (1993). Variant cytochrome P450 CYP2D6 allelic frequencies in Parkinson's disease. Am J Med Genet;339:911-922.

Lazzarini A, Myers RH, Zimmerman TR, Mark MH, Golbe LI, Sage ÊÊJI, Johnson WG, Duvoisin RC (1994). A clinical genetic study of Parkinson's disease: evidence for dominant transmission. Neurology; 44: 499-506.

Maraganore DM, Harding AE, Marsden CD (1991). A clinical and genetic study of familial Parkinson's disease. Movement Disord; 6: 205-211.

Maraganore DM, Muenter DM (1995). Personal communications.

Mjönes H. (1949), Paralysis agitans. A clinical genetic study. Acta Psychiatr Neurol Scand. 25(Suppl 54): 1-95.

Muenter MD, Howard FM, Okazaki H, Forno LS, Kish SJ, Hornykiewicz O (1986). A familial Parkinson-dementia syndrome. [Abstract] Neurology; 36 (Suppl 1):115.

Plante-Bordeneuve V, Davis MB, Maraganore DM et al. (1994). Tyrosine hydroxylase polymorphism in familial and sporadic Parkinson's disease. Mov Disord;9:337-339.

Ross CA, McInnis MG, Margolis RL, Shi-Hua L. Genes with triplet repeats: candidate mediators of neuropsychiatric disorders. TINS 1993;16:254-260.

Spellman GG (1962). Report of familial cases of Parkinsonism. Journal of the American Medical Association; 179:160-162.

Tanaka H, Ishakawa A, Ginns EI et al. (1991). Linkage analysis of juvenile Parkinsonism to tyrosine hydroxylase gene locus on chromosome 11. Neurology;41:719-722.

Waters CH, Miller CA (1994). Autosomal dominant Lewy body Parkinsonism in a four-generation family. Ann Neurol; 35: 59-64.

Wszolek ZK, Cordes M, Calne DB, Muenter MD, Cordes I, Pfeifer RF. (1993). Heredit Šrer Morbus Parkinson: Bericht uber drei Familiien mit autosomal-dominantem Erbang. Nervenarzt; 64: 331-335.

Wszolek ZK, Pfeiffer B, Fulgham JR, Parisi JE, Thompson RM, Uitti RJ, Calne DB, Pfeiffer RF (1995). Western Nebraska family (family D) with autosomal dominant Parkinsonism, Neurology;45:502-505.

PET Applications to Surgical Treatment of Parkinson's Disease

David Eidelberg

This paper will focus on the nature of modern PET applications to the study of surgical treatments of Parkinsonism. Most people appreciate that in Parkinson's disease the lesion itself involves a loss of dopaminergic cells in the pars compacta of the substantia nigra. Fluorodopa, a radiolabeled analog of Sinemet which can be given to patients and imaged with PET, is useful for gauging the severity of Parkinsonism. This tracer accumulates in the dopamine containing brain cells emanating from the substantia nigra to the striatum. In Parkinson's disease these cells degenerate and one sees a deterioration in the distribution of this tracer. PET becomes an objective means of assessing disease severity. Patients with the earliest stages of their disease, who demonstrate mild signs only on one side of the body, can be discriminated from their normal age-matched counterparts by using fluorodopa and PET. This method can also be applied to the study of fetal transplants for Parkinson's disease. We have found that in some patients the fluorodopa remains more or less reduced in the area of the putamen for up to 18 months after implantation. Indeed, one may not see a change in the fluorodopa at first. The period of time for the implantation to take place may vary quite a bit between patients. We have recently scanned someone who had been transplanted 9-1/2 months ago and found an increase of approximately 10-15% in uptake, particularly in the area which was implanted in the posterior part of the putamen. The critical point here is not so much that the change is ob-

David Eidelberg, MD, is Director, Neurological PET and Movement Disorders Program, Department of Neurology, North Shore University Hospital, Manhasset and Associate Professor of Neurology, Cornell University Medical College, New York, NY.

[Haworth co-indexing entry note]: "PET Applications to Surgical Treatment of Parkinson's Disease." Eidelberg, David. Co-published simultaneously in *Loss, Grief & Care* (The Haworth Press, Inc.) Vol. 8, No. 3/4, 2000, pp. 55-57; and: *Parkinson's Disease and Quality of Life* (ed: Côté et al.) The Haworth Press, Inc., 2000, pp. 55-57. Single or multiple copies of this article are available for a fee from The Haworth Document Delivery Service [1-800-342-9678, 9:00 a.m. - 5:00 p.m. (EST). E-mail address: getinfo@haworthpressinc.com].

served on PET but that it correlates with the clinical improvement that the patient experiences. Thus, PET is a useful means of validating the biological function of the implant. We also use PET for looking at new drugs that may serve as adjuncts to levodopa. Their efficacy in increasing levodopa accumulation in the brain can be assessed by these methods of positron emission tomography.

To move on to the area of glucose metabolic abnormalities in Parkinson's disease. What one sees at the earliest stages of Parkinsonism is an increase in glucose utilization localized to the area of the pallidum. The issue of pallidal hypermetabolism turns out to be critical to the understanding of the pathophysiology of the illness and also for planning surgical interventions. Not every patient exhibits this hypermetabolism. We found that cohorts of patients, perhaps accounting for as many as a third of patients diagnosed clinically as having PD fail to respond in a sustained way to levodopa. A number of these patients have other illnesses such as striatronigral degeneration which can be demonstrated with glucose PET. We have also used methods of network analysis to understand the relationships between brain regions and their function rather than their anatomy. In Parkinsonism, there is a hyperactivity of inhibitory networks emanating from the lentiform nucleus going into the thalamus and then ultimately a shut-off of motor cortical areas. We found that network expression in Parkinsonian patients also correlates quite closely with their disease severity. A specific network appears to be a constant signature of the disease and its expression in individual subjects. The greater the expression of this network the more severe the Parkinsonism. We find that this network can be used to differentiate typical Parkinson's disease, i.e., Sinemet responsive patients, from their drug-resistant counterparts. Additionally, small asymmetries in glucose metabolism favoring the side contralateral to the clinical involvement can be used in early diagnosis. This method allows us to identify drug resistant patients at the earliest stages of the illness.

We believe that a coherent strategy in imaging is needed for diagnosis and for assessing therapy. Our findings suggest that the pallido-thalamic network may actually become more accentuated in the course of Parkinsonism and that it may be an apt target for surgery. In addition, we have also been involved in pallidotomy research. Our interest has been to determine whether surgically lesioning the pallidum had some benefit on abnormal brain metabolism. We learned that the improvement that people experienced after pallidotomy appeared to correlate rather well with their preoperative hypermetabolism in that area of the brain. The patients that were more abnormal to begin with and had a hot area were those that actually did better following pallidotomy. Conversely, those patients that had striatonigral degeneration who have a cool area because of another neurodegenerative process do not improve as much. We have also learned that the thalamus is being hyperinhibited by the pallidum in this illness and that both pallidum and thalamus may be appropriate sites for surgery. If one places the lesion in the pallidum the abnormal thalamic hypermetabolism decreases. This change in metabolism correlated with the percent improvement that they experienced. Thus, pallidotomy can influence brain activity in key brain regions that are very far away from the surgical site. Our studies with PET show that this technique may not only be helpful in diagnosing Parkinson's disease, but may have considerable benefit in assessing new surgical therapies.

Can Your Insurance Manage
the Demands of a Chronic Illness?

Bruce J. Freshman

The various financial problems which face people today are compounded when a person, or a family member, develops a chronic disease. Financial plans must be rethought and redone, while some of the basic insurance products which accompany these plans either become scarce, limited, unobtainable, or more expensive.

Private insurance companies are, like any other type of business, profit motivated. Their objective is to insure healthy people, and, through careful underwriting (the process of determining the individual risk based on health and occupation) approve those who represent the smallest claim risk. Once approved, if the individual does become ill, injured, or dies, then the insurance company abides by the contract and pays the necessary claims.

Fortunately, the advancements in medical science and technology have dramatically increased longevity and recovery. On the downside, the cost for these procedures has skyrocketed. This is most apparent in the health or major medical fields. Take a typical family of four, over a 30 year span they will experience with the usual medical problems: broken bones, hernias, appendix, tonsils, emergency room visits, childbirth, auto accidents, etc.

Now take the same family but now one member has a pre-existing chronic condition . . . more frequent doctor visits, more specialized doctors, medication, physical therapy, new vaccines, new treatments, etc. The cost can be staggering . . . and it's on-going.

For those with chronic pre-existing conditions who work for 'large' companies, you have a reprieve with group major medical health insurance. The cost is minimal compared to individual coverage. Usually a person cannot be

Bruce J. Freshman, CLU, is affiliated with P.F.R. Planning, Inc., New York, NY.

[Haworth co-indexing entry note]: "Can Your Insurance Manage the Demands of a Chronic Illness?" Freshman, Bruce J. Co-published simultaneously in *Loss, Grief & Care* (The Haworth Press, Inc.) Vol. 8, No. 3/4, 2000, pp. 59-64; and: *Parkinson's Disease and Quality of Life* (ed: Côté et al.) The Haworth Press, Inc., 2000, pp. 59-64. Single or multiple copies of this article are available for a fee from The Haworth Document Delivery Service [1-800-342-9678, 9:00 a.m. - 5:00 p.m. (EST). E-mail address: getinfo@haworthpressinc.com].

59

singled out and charged more since the risk is spread throughout the group as a whole.

Unfortunately, laws and conversion privileges in group health insurance are not uniform throughout the country. For this reason, obtain a copy of the group benefits booklet, *and read it carefully!* The booklet will contain all insurance provided to each employee by the company; e.g., major medical insurance, long and short term disability, term life insurance, conversion privileges and restrictions, social security benefits, and Workman's Compensation. If one or more types of insurance are not mentioned, then it is probably not provided . . . *but double-check.*

Concerning group major medical, find out how much the deductible and co-insurance payments are. The deductible is paid out-of-pocket once per plan year by each covered person with a maximum dollar amount, or two or three deductibles can be charged per family. If the family pays co-insurance, out-of-pocket expenses are capped. "Covered Persons" are the employee and his/her insured dependents. Also, see if there are cost containment features, prescription cards, and if pre-authorizations or second opinions are required for surgery? If clarification is needed, ask the benefits department personnel. If the answer is still unsatisfactory, call the insurance company directly. People need to identify themselves to the insurance company through their group membership number.

In most instances, when leaving a group plan, it can be converted to an individual plan simply by filling out a form. If there is this conversion privilege, it cannot be declined. Also, if a person leaves a company having twenty or more employees, the company must extend the group coverage to that person for a period of 18 months . . . *and 18 months only.* This extension is provided by the C.O.B.R.A. Law, and was designed to protect people between jobs. The individual has to pay the full premium plus a small charge, but it is well worth it.

To keep down costs on an individual plan, choose a high deductible in addition to a high coinsurance feature. Tailor your health insurance plan to cover those costs which you cannot cover out-of-pocket. Also, try to set up your own private side fund which, in later years, can help cover the cost of high deductibles and coinsurance.

Whether in a group health plan or an individual plan, once approved or already in a plan, a person cannot be terminated from the plan, *no matter what illness he/she has.*

If one has no coverage and develops a chronic illness, private companies will not insure the person unless he/she joins a large company. But there is an alternative: Blue Cross/Blue Shield. Check with the BC/BS in a specific state. Usually no one can be declined coverage. It should be noted, though, that they do impose an eleven month exclusion clause for all pre-existing conditions, after which time a person is fully covered. Three basic complaints about BC/BS is their telephone lines are constantly busy, the same representative is not available each time, and their maximum lifetime coverage is one million dollars. True as these may be, their representatives are courteous and knowledgeable, and the coverage is good. Again, for additional information, call a local BC/BS chapter. Know that BC/BS is seeking increases on a continuous basis, and in some states they are attempting to divide high risk groups from standard groups (so far they have been denied).

Having continuous uninterrupted coverage for a chronic condition is possible with careful planning. It is called *'piggy-backing' or 'double coverage.'* This is how it works! Blue Cross/Blue Shield has an eleven month exclusion for all pre-existing conditions before there is full coverage. Assuming an individual is presently covered, but plans to leave his/her job for whatever reason in the next year. He/she should sign up for BC/BS now even though he/she is already covered under the present plan. This might require double health premiums, but after 11 months the individual will be fully covered from the 'Blues' and can then drop the old coverage. This can also be done on C.O.B.R.A. . . . just remember the 18 month limit.

MEDICARE/MEDICAID/MEDIGAP

Medicare and *Medicaid* are going through constant changes with no end in sight. We are also approaching the 'baby boomer' generation and, ironically, this large generation had the fewest children. For those in their forties, it will be one of the largest generations being supported tax-wise by one of the smallest generations. The outcome is anyone's guess!

Medicare is only for those 65 years old. It is standardized throughout the country, and one cannot be turned down for coverage. An individual must apply for Medicare 6 months before turning age 65, and the premium is automatically taken out of the Social Security checks (the government takes no chances!). *Part-A* covers hospitalization and is mandatory. *Part-B* is optional and covers surgery.

Medigap policies cover those costs not covered at all, or insufficiently, by Medicare. Medigap policies wrap around Parts A and B of Medicare, so Part B of Medicare must be taken before enrolling in a Medigap plan. New York State standardized ten Medigap plans concerning basic coverage (differences in premiums is based on the extras available). Also, effective May 1, 1992 in New York State, any Medicare beneficiary 65 or older has six months in which to obtain Medicare supplement insurance regardless of medical condition. However, individuals may still be subject to a six month waiting period for coverage of pre-existing conditions. This 'open enrollment' period to apply for Medicare supplemental coverage begins with the first month in which the person 65 or older enrolls for Medicare Part-B benefits.

People should check with their State Insurance Department to verify one way or another if this is available where they live. If it is not, or if the opportunity has passed, they should make sure their primary physician refers them only to those doctors who take assignment (which means the doctor will accept Medicare allowable charges as his total fee).

Medicaid is the federal health program for lower income families, and you do not have to be age 65 to be eligible. There are volunteers in many hospitals who specialize in teaching patients about Medicare and Medicaid and assist them in filling out the forms. These volunteers know all the forms and qualifications and guide people through this maze. They are truly remarkable, knowledgeable, and friendly people who are there only to help.

DISABILITY INSURANCE

Disability Insurance replaces lost earned income due to illness or injury. If long term disability is offered at work . . . *take it! Take all that is available!* Unlike health insurance which can be converted to an individual plan, usually there is no such privilege for disability. The common group disability plan pays 60-70% of salary, bonuses not included, until age 65. This plan can be offset by Social Security and Workman's Compensation.

Very few insurance companies offer disability to people with pre-existing conditions since all they would be inheriting is an ongoing claim!

If disability is not offered at work, employees are still covered by Workman's Compensation (this is limited to on the job accidents) and Social Security Disability (over 70% of those who apply for disability benefits are turned down).

LIFE INSURANCE/TERM INSURANCE

Another way to help compensate for the lack of disability coverage are certain types of life insurance. Life insurance is one of the few insurance products still available for people with health problems (mainly because everyone only dies once). Life insurance represents the same uniqueness for everyone; it creates an immediate liquid, in some cases, tax-free, estate to insure the continued uninterrupted lifestyle for one's family. Another valuable feature is the accumulating cash value. This increasing cash value belongs to the policy owner and is available at any time. This represents an ongoing source of ready cash for medical emergencies, to cover high deductibles or coinsurance, or a self insuring fund in times of disability.

Attached to some health plans is term insurance which can range from minimal amounts to higher amounts based on income and/or bonus. Always take advantage of this option since, at the initial stage, there are no medical requirements.

Upon leaving a company, the life insurance is convertible to an individual policy with no medical requirements. The downside is that this conversion is only available upon leaving, and only for the amount of term insurance in the health plan. Also, the premium will be based on the individual person's age at conversion. Since there is no cash value with term insurance, many years can pass during which one could have been building a tax deferred fund for oneself.

At all times, taking out cash value life insurance at a young age makes sense. Aside from the years of increasing cash, once a life insurance policy is issued, they only one who can break this contract is the policy holder. And, regardless of health, the premiums will never increase over the life of the contract.

Although there are many life insurance companies, only a handful specialize in *"impaired risks"* (individuals who have chronic health problems). Not only do these companies offer a better chance of being approved, but the cost factor can be significantly lower from these specialized companies. The impaired risk companies will consider persons who have been rejected by other insurance companies. These companies underwrite on an individual basis with standard limits applying.

OTHER FINANCIAL OPTIONS

Besides insurance products, there are a host of other financial products available without regard to health. One of the most popular is the mutual fund. A mutual fund is where a large number of people pool their money together under the investment strategy of the fund manager. And just as everyone's money is pooled, so are a variety of stocks. This diminishes the volatility of owning individual stocks.

There are also money market funds, bond funds, sector funds, etc. Every year, magazines such as *Forbes, Money,* and *U.S. News & World Report* list the top funds and/or family of funds. Annuities are another tax-deferred investment vehicle. Some annuities incorporate mutual funds inside the contract for even greater growth potential. A year ago the Federal Government attempted to do away with the tax-deferral status of annuities but it did not pass. It's a good bet that they will try again, and hopefully any money deposited before the change would be 'grandfathered,' exempt from the new law. Stocks, bonds, real estate, and mutual funds are good investments over the long haul. But, like everything else, talk to an expert who is known and trusted in the field.

CLOSING COMMENT

In conclusion, having a chronic condition does require extra planning, but the first step should always be to know exactly what benefits are provided through one's job, and to take full advantage of them. The next step is the same as everyone else's . . . always pay oneself first. No matter how little, the first bill to pay is to oneself whether it be in the form of mutual funds, life insurance premiums, bank accounts, stocks, bonds, or under the pillow. The key is to start early and be consistent.

Maximizing Independence:
Occupational Therapy Intervention
for Patients with Parkinson's Disease

Glen Gillen

Occupational therapy intervention for patients with Parkinson's disease is aimed at promoting wellness by assuring that the patient is functioning at his/her maximum potential in terms of the occupational roles that he/she fills. Occupational roles can be categorized into the areas of activities of daily living (i.e., dressing, feeding, transferring, bed mobility, etc.), work (including family and home management), and leisure. It is the goal of occupational therapy, from the onset of disease, that patients resume and/or assume new occupational roles. Because this disease progresses over a period of time, occupational therapy interventions will change depending on the level of dependence with which a patient presents. Therefore, it is recommended that a patient be evaluated by an occupational therapist at various intervals throughout the course of the disease (Pedretti). This article will outline common problem areas seen in patients with Parkinson's disease, review how these problems interfere with functional independence, and finally provide examples of occupational therapy intervention and treatment techniques. The most common symptoms seen in patients with Parkinson's disease patients are bradykinesia, akinesia, tremor, rigidity ("cogwheel" or "leadpipe"), and postural control alterations (Melnick). These symptoms have a variety of detrimental effects on activities of daily living, in terms of purposeful upper extremity movement patterns (buttoning, managing liquids on a spoon, etc.)

Glen Gillen, MPA, OTR, is Supervisor of Inpatient Rehabilitation, New York Presbyterian Hospital and Instructor in Clinical Occupational Therapy, College of Physicians and Surgeons, Columbia University, New York, NY 10003.

[Haworth co-indexing entry note]: "Maximizing Independence: Occupational Therapy Intervention for Patients with Parkinson's Disease." Gillen, Glen. Co-published simultaneously in Loss, Grief & Care (The Haworth Press, Inc.) Vol. 8, No. 3/4, 2000, pp. 65-67; and: Parkinson's Disease and Quality of Life (ed: Côté et al.) The Haworth Press, Inc., 2000, pp. 65-67. Single or multiple copies of this article are available for a fee from The Haworth Document Delivery Service [1-800-342-9678, 9:00 a.m. - 5:00 p.m. (EST). E-mail address: getinfo@haworthpressinc.com].

and total body functional movement patterns such as sit to stand, rolling, supine to sit, etc.

Parkinson's disease patients begin experiencing upper extremity dysfunction early on in the course of the disease. Initial problem areas usually center around activities involving fine motor coordination. Writing is a common problem area. As this skill become impaired, occupational therapy intervention is indicated to evaluate for and fabricate adaptive writing devices. As micrography becomes increasingly present, a typewriter is beneficial for both work tasks and continued social correspondence, in many cases.

Manipulation of feeding utensils is a common complaint and has both social implications (the embarrassment of food spillage) and self-esteem issues (infantilization issues of having to be fed by a caretaker). Adaptive feeding equipment is indicated in these cases to compensate for dyscontrol of hand to mouth patterns. Adaptive equipment may include built-up handles on utensils, rocker/roller knives for one-handed cutting, no-slip surfaces for plates, and lidded cups to prevent spillage.

Bradykinesia and tremors are the most frequent motor control deficits that interfere in dressing activities. Dressing tasks can become excruciatingly slow and tedious for patients with Parkinson's disease. In these cases, an occupational therapist will assess the effectiveness of adaptive dressing techniques and prescribe adaptive dressing equipment if necessary. Adaptive equipment is designed to decrease the time involved in dressing, compensate for fine motor coordination deficits, and/or compensate for decreased trunk range of motion involved in lower extremity dressing. During a dressing evaluation, the following must be taken into consideration: the role of the caretaker, the optimal positions for energy conservation, ease of task completion, and safety precautions.

It is worthwhile at this point to discuss caretaker roles. Because of the increased time associated with self-care tasks, it is common for caretakers to "overassist," and in essence, foster dependence. There are many variables that must be taken into consideration when training individuals to assist with self-care. How important is it to the patient to carry out these tasks independently? Will the patient have enough energy for the rest of the day's activities if he/she performs these tasks independently but with increased time and effort? How frustrating are these tasks to the patient? The goal is to achieve a balance between activities and rest while providing optimal opportunities for patients to perform independently and enhance self-esteem needs.

In patients with advanced disease, postural control and mobility deficits may interfere to the point that a patient will require a wheelchair. The proper wheelchair prescription must take into consideration a variety of factors. A proper seating system may prevent further deformity and/or compensate for fixed deformities (traditionally kyphosis with resulting head/neck flexion).

Patients that continue to sit in a flexed posture have a decreased vital capacity, a tendency to drool, and have limited social interaction secondary to poor eye contact. The proper seat cushion must be prescribed to prevent skin breakdown and to control asymmetry of the pelvis. Finally, the proper wheelchair must encourage functional independence in terms of independent wheelchair propulsion.

Occupational therapy treatment will also focus on prescribing a home exercise program. A home exercise program should be built into the patient's daily activities. The program should focus on the maintenance of upper extremity and trunk range of motion, stretching, coordination, as well as maintaining general endurance and activity tolerance. A home exercise program must be geared to a patient's present functional status and include activities that are meaningful to the patient. An example of a home exercise program for a higher level patient may be as simple as organizing kitchen cabinets. This task encourages shoulder range of motion, trunk extension, various hand patterns, and overhead activities without being rote exercise.

In some cases, a critical intervention of occupational therapy is a home evaluation. This evaluation will allow the therapist, patient, and family to choose bathroom equipment (grab bars, tub seats, and commodes) which considers safety factors while maximizing independence. It will allow the therapist to point out potential fall areas such as throw rugs and electrical cords, as well as give suggestions to change the home environment to suit the patient's level of function.

Finally, in terms of intervention, an occupational therapist should evaluate a patient when they are benefitting most from their medication, and when the dose is wearing off, since functional status may be dramatically different. In this way, the therapist, patient, and family can decide when it is optimal to perform various activities and when to build rest patterns into the day.

REFERENCES

Melnick, M.E. 1990. "Basal Ganglia Disorders: Metabolic, Hereditary, and Genetic Disorders in Adults." In D.A. Umphred, ed. *Neurological Rehabilitation.* St. Louis: C.V. Mosby Co. pp. 559-568.

Pedretti, L.W. 1990. *Occupational Therapy: Practice Skills for Physical Dysfunction.* St. Louis: C.V. Mosby Co.

Brain Tissue Donation
in Research on Parkinsonism

James E. Goldman

This paper addresses some important questions regarding the value of brain donation in Parkinson's research. What do we do with brain tissues and why are they valuable to all of us? Despite the advances in our understanding of the basic pathophysiology of many neurodegenerative diseases there is plenty we still do not know. Much of the necessary research requires the use of human brain tissue. The now well known classic features of Parkinson's disease is the depletion of neurons in the substantia nigra. Neuromelanin contain neurons in the nigra and they contain eosinophilic inclusions that were described many, many years ago and are now called Lewy bodies. There has been some work by the British Columbia group that illustrates the number of cells in the substantia nigra. The determination of cell number could only be arrived at through the examination of human brain tissue.

The investigators took a block of tissue containing a human substantia nigra and cut it into very thin sections and counted the number of neurons in each section of nigra. We know from this study and from a number of other studies, that we all lose neurons in this region of the brain as we grow older. However, we also know, again from autopsy studies, that the number of neurons lost in the brains of patients with Parkinson's disease and other forms of nigral degeneration (not just idiopathic Parkinson's disease) is far, far greater in the Parkinson brain than as result from aging. These are classical sorts of studies, and it may be asked what more do we need to know? The main question still remains. Although we know something about the pathology of Parkinson's disease and the neuronal loss in Parkinson's disease, we do

---

James E. Goldman, MD, PhD, is Professor of Pathology, College of Physicians and Surgeons, Columbia University and Director, Division of Neuropathy, New York Presbyterian Hospital, New York, NY.

[Haworth co-indexing entry note]: "Brain Tissue Donation in Research on Parkinsonism." Goldman, James E. Co-published simultaneously in *Loss, Grief & Care* (The Haworth Press, Inc.) Vol. 8, No. 3/4, 2000, pp. 69-71; and: *Parkinson's Disease and Quality of Life* (ed: Côté et al.) The Haworth Press, Inc., 2000, pp. 69-71. Single or multiple copies of this article are available for a fee from The Haworth Document Delivery Service [1-800-342-9678, 9:00 a.m. - 5:00 p.m. (EST). E-mail address: getinfo@haworthpress inc.com].

not understand why those neurons are lost. Thus, the central question is: what's killing certain subsets of neurons? I might add that this is not just a question in Parkinson's disease research these days, but a central and focal question in research in all neurodegenerative diseases, including Alzheimer's disease, Pick's disease, a number of the Parkinson plus syndromes such as progressive supranuclear palsy and cortical basal degeneration and others. As Susan Calne has said, there is only a limited amount of work that we can do on the biochemistry and molecular biology of these problems in the living brain. For the important current and future studies, we require fresh and frozen central nervous system tissue, obtained at autopsy. For the last several years, we have maintained a large and growing tissue bank at Columbia Presbyterian Medical Center under the auspices of the Parkinson's Disease Foundation and NIH grants that support our research in Alzheimer's disease, Parkinson's disease, stroke and other age related neurodegenerative diseases. We receive brain tissue from autopsies that we do at the hospital and from patients who die in other hospitals or nursing homes, or even at home. At Presbyterian Hospital we try to remove brains within a few hours, if possible, because some of the biochemical functions and molecular components of the central nervous system begin to degenerate after death and if one waits too long, some of these functions (such as enzymes and mitochondrial oxidation that a lot of investigators are interested in) will have disappeared. So a rapid autopsy is very important. The other thing that is really required is that the fresh tissue be removed quickly and frozen quickly. As Susan Calne has said, the actual removal of the brain is not difficult and really only takes a few minutes. It is not a disfiguring process in the least. We routinely remove the brain, including the brainstem (that's critical because of loss of brainstem function in Parkinson's disease) and we fix some of the tissues so we can look at the cellular pathology and examine tissue for nigral cell loss and Lewy bodies. We also slice half of the brain, freeze the slices quickly and keep them in a very low temperature freezer. The low temperature will preserve a lot of the basic metabolic machinery. We keep detailed records of the patient and pathology records (the neuropathology report). We make this tissue available to investigators who have research programs that require the use of human tissue and we have sent the tissue to many of our colleagues at Columbia and to a number of laboratories around North America, Canada, Europe and Japan. Tissue banks represent invaluable resources. As our knowledge of these diseases increases, there always seems to be, every five or ten years or, hopefully, at shorter intervals than that, new ways of looking at tissue. The frozen tissue constitutes a resource that is available for years and years and can be returned to again and again as new findings require.

There is another difficult issue to be discussed. Why does there seem to be in many people's minds difficulty with the idea of the autopsy? Resistance to autopsies comes from physicians and nurses and other health care professionals as well as people who are not in the health care business. There seem to be a number of reasons for this resistance. First, the idea that now that we have PET scanning and sophisticated clinical evaluations, we know everything about a disease and thus there is nothing additional to learn from an autopsy is frankly not in the least true. There is a great deal that we still need to learn about these diseases and that we can only learn from tissue examination. Secondly, as I mentioned, the autopsy itself is not a disfiguring process. We have long, long experience in performing post-mortem examinations. There are some who have religious or ethical principles which argue against autopsies and will not be discussing those issues in this piece. Third, I have a comment particularly for family members of Parkinson patients. Despite the advances in our understanding of these diseases, our final diagnosis really rests in many cases with neuropathology. It is perhaps less true of idiopathic Parkinson's than it is of some of these so-called Parkinson plus syndromes, but even for Parkinson's disease, because of individual variations from person to person, it can be very difficult to be one-hundred percent certain. I think that we sometimes cannot be one-hundred percent certain even after an autopsy, in rare conditions, but there is still a lot that we can tell you about what happened to a family member. A clear diagnosis is particularly important for diseases in which there is a prominent genetic component.

Lesion Surgery for Parkinson's Disease: Practical Aspects of New Developments

Robert R. Goodman

This chapter will focus on presenting a neurosurgeon's perspective on the practical aspects of performing surgical lesions, or implanting brain stimulators, in an attempt to improve the symptoms of Parkinson's disease. Thalamotomy has been the most widely performed surgery for Parkinson's disease, dating back more than 35 years now. Thalamotomy has been very effective in alleviating one of the symptoms of Parkinson's, tremor. Recently a better understanding of the neural circuitry involved in Parkinson's and review of the early experience with pallidotomy has led to an increasing application of lesions in the globus pallidus (pallidotomy) which has helped patients with Parkinson's disease. It is important to note that pallidotomy has the potential to improve the most disabling features of Parkinson's disease and also alleviate tremor in many patients. Parkinson's is a slowly progressive disease that eventually causes severe functional impairment. Prior to the availability of L-Dopa and other medications, Parkinson's patients rapidly became disabled and a variety of brain lesions were performed in an attempt to alleviate symptoms. L-Dopa and other therapies dramatically changed the approach to Parkinson's disease.

Medications greatly improved the symptoms of rigidity, limited movement (bradykinesia) and gait difficulty. However, tremor was not responsive to the medications. Thalamotomy has been used throughout the last 35 years to alleviate tremor in those relatively rare patients who are disabled by this symptom. Unfortunately, Parkinson's is a progressive disease and although medication is dramatically effective, eventually symptoms progress and med-

Robert R. Goodman, MD, PhD, is Assistant Professor of Neurological Surgery, College of Physicians and Surgeons, Columbia University, New York, NY 10032.

[Haworth co-indexing entry note]: "Lesion Surgery for Parkinson's Disease: Practical Aspects of New Developments." Goodman, Robert R. Co-published simultaneously in *Loss, Grief & Care* (The Haworth Press, Inc.) Vol. 8, No. 3/4, 2000, pp. 73-78; and: *Parkinson's Disease and Quality of Life* (ed: Côté et al.) The Haworth Press, Inc., 2000, pp. 73-78. Single or multiple copies of this article are available for a fee from The Haworth Document Delivery Service [1-800-342-9678, 9:00 a.m. - 5:00 p.m. (EST). E-mail address: getinfo@haworthpressinc.com].

ications fail to prevent severe disability. Progressive disability is due to worsening of the so called "negative symptoms" of Parkinson's, rigidity, bradykinesia and loss of balance and particularly the development of erratic fluctuations in the response to L-Dopa treatment. A neurosurgeon in Sweden, Lauri Laitenin, recently reported his experience with ventral posterior lesions in the globus pallidus for Parkinson's patients with these disabling symptoms. His interest in this lesion arose from a review of patients who had received similar lesions by Dr. Laitenin's professor, Professor Leksell, more than 20 years earlier.

The symptom of tremor must be considered separately from the other symptoms of Parkinson's disease. Extensive experience with lesions in the thalamus has demonstrated that this approach can be very effective in the treatment of disabling tremor that fails to respond to medication. The same lesion is quite effective for patients that have the condition termed Essential Tremor, without Parkinson's disease. Pallidotomy is a lesion of a different anatomical target at a different level of the altered circuitry of Parkinson's disease. The details of the circuitry and importance of the globus pallidus are presented in Dr. DeLong's chapter. This chapter will focus on selection of appropriate patients for surgery, practical issues involved in the performance of these surgeries and the results of surgery.

As mentioned above, the patients with disabling tremor that remains uncontrollable with medication are candidates for the thalamotomy procedure. Candidates for the pallidotomy procedure are less easily defined. Further experience will be required before it is clear which patients are appropriate candidates. At this time, it seems that patients disabled by erratic fluctuations in their response to medication are the best candidates for the pallidotomy procedure. The procedure appears to improve response to medication. Patients continue to take similar doses of L-Dopa and other medications, but are less bothered by the symptoms of rigidity, bradykinesia, gait difficulty, "offs," and drug-induced dyskinesias. Pallidotomy also has been reported to improve tremor in many patients. Thus, patients who are still responding to L-Dopa may be the best candidates for pallidotomy, but patients who no longer have even brief periods of good motor function may not be benefitted by the pallidotomy procedure.

Thalamotomy and pallidotomy procedures are in many ways technically quite similar to each other. Both procedures involve the placement of a very precise and fairly small lesion in the brain. Imaging studies are improving at a dramatic pace, but as yet do not allow us to precisely identify the exact target areas in the brain. Surgical approaches involve the use of imaging to bring a lesioning electrode (generally about 1 mm in diameter) to within several millimeters of the ultimate target for lesioning. The precise placement of a lesion is then adjusted by using physiological techniques to confirm appropriate targeting. One method for doing this utilizes the lesioning electrode to pass an electrical current and thus stimulate the brain area. The exact response to stimulation (either sensation reported by the patient or movement that can be seen) can be used to confirm the electrode location. Many centers are using a different technique, which may allow more precise identification of the brain area. This is by using a so-called micro-electrode initially, which permits the recording of nerve activity from individual neurons. This type of information can provide much more precise determination of the local brain anatomy. This can permit a positive identification of the target area before changing the micro to a macro-electrode to allow stimulation and then lesioning.

Although the goals of various surgeries are basically the same, the techniques used to achieve these goals vary significantly. The initial stage involves combining imaging with a frame secured to the patient's head. Early surgeries used ventriculography, which involved injection of dye into the ventricle (clear brain fluid) and then x-rays of the skull. Other techniques used the CAT scan alone or in combination with ventriculography. These approaches can allow accurate identification of two important internal landmarks in the brain, the anterior and posterior commissures. Atlases of the brain have been created in relation to these commissures. The relationship of various brain structures to the commissure varies somewhat between different individuals. The atlases would allow a close approximation of the target area once the location of the commissures is known precisely. The specific anatomy of any one particular patient is determined by using a macro-electrode for brain stimulation or micro-electrode for the monitoring of individual brain cell activity, as described above. Thus, imaging brings the electrode within several millimeters of the desired target and stimulation and recording techniques allow refinement of this to within less than 1 mm of the desired target.

Many centers are beginning to utilize MRI to target lesions, because it may allow improved accuracy for the initial placement of the electrode. The MRI allows much better visualization of the internal anatomy of the brain. It has been technically difficult to use the MRI in conjunction with the stereotactic frames that are needed to guide the electrodes in these lesioning procedures. The MRI produces a slightly distorted image and this significantly impairs accuracy in stereotactic procedures. Some techniques are not able to overcome the drawback of this distortion. At Columbia we have been working on the application of a computer work station to allow the use of MRI to accurately guide these procedures. The computer allows us to take a routine MRI (obtained without any device secured to the patients' head) and merge it with the CAT scan obtained with a stereotactic frame secured to the patient's head. This procedure eliminates the distortion of the MRI and allows us to achieve the accuracy of the CAT scan with the internal detail available on the MRI. The ability to use the MRI accurately has significantly enhanced the lesioning procedures. The MRI allows us to see a detail of brain structures that is very close to that which is available with the stereotactic atlases of the human brain itself. Also, the MRI allows us to view the brain in more than one orientation, greatly increasing our ability to choose the correct target and trajectory for initial electrode placement.

Improved imaging has improved our ability to reach the desired brain target, however, it is still important to confirm the location with physiology before lesioning. Some error of computation, mechanical shifting of the device or movement of the brain between the acquisition of imaging and the placement of the electrode can introduce an error. The stimulation studies or micro electrode recording studies are needed to precisely define the target area. An attempt is made to identify the center of the desired target. The lesions created are typically 3 to 4 millimeters in diameter and 3 to 8 millimeters in length. The lesions are often over 70 cubic millimeters in volume. This must always be kept in mind when considering the accuracy needed for targeting. The micro-electrode provides more accurate identification of brain anatomy than does the macro-electrode, but after extremely precise mapping with the micro-electrode a rather massive lesion (in comparison) is created. The microelectrode technique demands a much greater investment in equipment, time of operation and number of brain penetrations with electrodes. It is important that we be certain that the improved accuracy leads to an improved outcome if we are to require this approach in addition to the macro-electrode/stimulation approach. The anatomy in the thalamus lends itself very well to characterization with the macro electrode/stimulation approach. In this area it is not clear that the micro-electrode significantly alters the lesion placement. To date, in the globus pallidus it is not yet clear that the anatomy will allow stimulation to adequately define the targeting. Positive identification of the globus pallidus with a micro-electrode may substantially improve our ability to accurately lesion the appropriate area and avoid injuring nearby non-targeted areas (see also Dr. DeLong's chapter regarding these issues).

Thalamotomies and pallidotomies are procedures that last from 1 to more than 8 hours, depending on the exact approach utilized. The patients remain awake and interactive throughout the procedure. At times, patients may be given sedation to help them tolerate certain uncomfortable portions of the operation. A stereotactic frame is secured to the head, imaging studies are obtained, and then the patient is brought to the operating room. In the operating room, a small area on the top of the head is shaved, a local anesthetic injected, a small incision is made and a small hole in the skull is created. Then, the stereotactic device allows guidance of electrodes to the desired targets. Recording studies, stimulation studies, and then, lesioning is carried out, much of which requires interaction with the patient. Improvement of the patient's condition is usually seen immediately upon creation of the lesion. The entire procedure is generally no more uncomfortable than a common dental procedure or a stereotactic brain biopsy, a relatively common brain operation.

Thalamotomy has been reported to achieve elimination of dramatic improvement of tremor in over 80 percent of patients. There is a small risk of recurrence of tremor over time following the procedure. As with any brain surgery, there is some risk involved. Large series of surgeries have been reported with an overall incidence of approximately 1 percent of serious complications. The single most serious risk from the procedure is hemorrhage and stroke. Lesioning can also cause altered speech, numbness or weakness. The incidence of these complications is *less* than 10 percent in most centers.

Results of pallidotomy for Parkinson's disease are more difficult to summarize. The experience with pallidotomy is more recent and differences in patient selection and technique of surgery makes it difficult to combine results from various surgical centers. The experience of Dr. Laitenin in Sweden suggests that 80 percent of patients significantly improve after pallidotomy. This improvement includes decrease of drug-induced involuntary movements, rigidity, bradykinesia and gait difficulty. Also, 80 percent of patients have been reported to have some improvement of tremor. A similar approximately 1 percent risk of stroke exists and a somewhat higher risk of loss of a portion of peripheral vision has been noted. More recent experience at surgical centers in the United States appears to be achieving similar, and possibly even more promising results.

Another approach to these same problems involves the implantation of a permanent brain stimulator into the same anatomical locations that are typically lesioned in these procedures. The objective of this approach is to place an electrode in place of creating a lesion. The procedure itself is in many ways similar to the lesion procedure, except that the electrode is left in place at the end of the procedure rather than using it to burn a small area of the brain. A more extensive procedure is required, because a device to generate an electrical current is placed under the skin and wires are passed under the skin to connect to the electrode in the brain. The theoretical advantage of this approach would be to allow reversible inactivation of the desired brain area. Thus, when the stimulator is on, the same area that would have been lesioned is now made inactive by the electrical current. That area can then regain its activity when the stimulator is turned off. This may eliminate some of the undesired side effects of lesioning, such as impairments of speech or vision. Certain negative aspects may apply to this procedure as well. The stimulator and its wires can develop mechanical difficulties that may require surgery for repair. In some cases, the brain may lose its responsiveness to the stimulation and either movement of the electrode or creation of a lesion with burning may be required to regain benefit. Also, implantation of such device carries a higher risk of infection than a lesion procedure. There has been substantial experience with these electrodes in Europe that has been quite promising. To date, this procedure is being carried out on an experimental basis in the United States and experience is somewhat limited. Only time will reveal whether stimulation is more advantageous than the traditional lesion procedures.

The paliidotomy procedure for Parkinson's disease appears to be a very exciting treatment for patients with disabling Parkinson's disease. Our new understanding of the brain circuitry involved in Parkinson's disease has combined with new technology for brain surgery to provide an exciting new alternative in the treatment of Parkinson's disease. It is important to remember that the intended result of brain lesions, based on our knowledge of the brain circuitry, is not always the proper explanation of the lesion's result. Empirical observations of lesion placement and effect on patients must be continuously scrutinized. Alternative explanations may exist for the observed results. The positive results obtained and risks involved with any procedure are the most important factors, although improvement of our understanding of brain functioning will likely lead to improvements of our surgical interventions.

Reviewing the Case
for an Environmental Cause
of Parkinson's Disease

Danielle Greene

INTRODUCTION

Parkinson's disease (PD) is a neurodegenerative disease that affects mobility and muscle control. Although this is a disorder that generally affects people over the age of 60, there is a subset of the disease called "early onset" PD that is usually detected in people between the ages of 40 and 60. The outward symptoms of PD include a stiffness of the body and facial expressions, tremors (usually of the hands), and difficulty in walking. Progression of the disease causes further loss of muscle control. Parkinsonians (the term for people affected by the disease) often experience difficulty in speaking as the disease progresses because these muscles become weak and they find themselves unable to project their voices as they finish their sentences.

PD was first discovered by James Parkinson in 1817 in Great Britain. Researchers still debate whether this is when the disease first appeared or if this was the first time a scientist was able to pull the disparate symptoms of the disease together into a diagnosis (Tanner and Langston, 1990). This will be a particularly relevant fact in the discussion of environmental causes.

It is now known that the symptoms of Parkinson's disease are caused by death of cells in the substantia nigra section of the brain. These cells produce dopamine which controls muscle movement. Most treatments for PD involve the prescription of drugs like Sinamet, Selegiline, and Bromocriptine, whose

Danielle Greene, MPH, is affiliated with the Joseph L. Moulman School of Public Health, Columbia University, New York, NY.

[Haworth co-indexing entry note]: "Reviewing the Case for an Environmental Cause of Parkinson's Disease." Greene, Danielle. Co-published simultaneously in *Loss, Grief & Care* (The Haworth Press, Inc.) Vol. 8, No. 3/4, 2000, pp. 79-85; and: *Parkinson's Disease and Quality of Life* (ed: Côté et al.) The Haworth Press, Inc., 2000, pp. 79-85. Single or multiple copies of this article are available for a fee from The Haworth Document Delivery Service [1-800-342-9678, 9:00 a.m. - 5:00 p.m. (EST). E-mail address: getinfo@haworthpressinc.com].

functions are to either add dopamine to the brain or increase the dopamine production of the surviving cells (UCSD School of Medicine Web Page on Parkinson's Disease). Many researchers believe it is the mitochondria of the cells that is malfunctioning and causing the dopamine-producing cells to die. It is also believed that this is the result of antioxidants and free oxygen radical production (interview with Dr. Côté, 1996; Langston, 1987).

The combination of symptoms identifying PD: bradykinesia (too much movement), rigidity (lack of movement), resting tremor, can be seen as a result of several disorders (Rajput, 1993). The three most common symptoms are often referred to as Parkinson's Syndrome or Parkinsonism. Some of these are caused by strokes, dementia, or certain drugs. The type of PD affecting the most people and to be discussed here is known as idiopathic PD, meaning cause unknown.

HYPOTHETICAL MECHANISMS
OF AN ENVIRONMENTAL AGENT

Examination of mortality data shows that mortality rates for PD increase with age (as do incidence rates). There does seem to be a cluster of deaths within the 75 to 84 year old category, after which the rate decreases (Schoenberg, 1987). It has also been observed that PD mortality "has remained relatively stable over time" in the U.S., England, and Wales (Schoenberg, 1987: 408). Studies show that the dopamine producing cells in the substantia nigra have a short life span naturally (interview with Dr. Côté, 1996). As all people age, they lose these cells. In people with PD, this reduction occurs more dramatically and earlier. Because of PD's prevalence among older individuals, it is believed that among the more elderly there is a tendency to misdiagnosis the signs of PD as simply a result of the normal aging process (Tanner, 1990). It is believed by some that everyone will develop PD if they live long enough (interview with Dr. Côté, 1996). Morbidity and mortality studies often undercount or miscount deaths from PD because it is not frequently listed as the underlying cause of death and is often not listed on the death certificate at all (Tanner, 1990). An example of this is one study which reported that PD was listed on the death certificate in 61 percent of the cases looked at but was listed as the cause of death in only 30 percent (Schulte, 1996).

Because of this data, several scientists propose that it is a combination of factors that cause PD. Tanner et al., in their 1987 review article report some authors believe that "PD may be the combined product of a neurotoxic environmental agent combined with normal aging" while others suggest "a heritable susceptibility to environmental toxins, leading to the development of PD if an appropriate toxin is environmentally present" (Tanner et al.,

1987: 419; Schoenberg, 1987). This could refer to an agent that speeds up the natural degeneration of the dopamine producing cells, a toxin that directly damages the dopamine producing cells, or that in certain people, there is a reaction to certain toxins which is detrimental to these specific cells.

Familial studies suggest that there is a greater likelihood of malfunctioning dopamine cells in related people (Tanner et al., 1987). This may be physiologically, not environmentally, induced. Parkinson's is generally believed to be familial but not directly inherited. First degree relatives of persons afflicted with PD have a "two fold increased risk" of acquiring the disease (interview with Dr. Côté, 1996). The typical pattern of inheritance is uncle to nephew or cousin. A parent and child both having PD is rare.

Several studies of twins have compared identical patterns and rates of aging and found different rates of developing PD (Tanner, 1990). These studies have been used as arguments against the genetic-cause or age-related cause theories. There is no known PD gene at this time. Dr. Lucien Côté, neurologist specializing in Parkinson's disease at Columbia-Presbyterian Medical Center, does not expect one to be found (interview with Dr. Côté, 1996). Dr. Paul Greene, another neurologist with a specialty in Parkinson's disease at Columbia-Presbyterian Medical Center, believes that the familial pattern of PD is suggestive of a dominant gene with penetrance. This means that, while only one affected gene is necessary to cause the disease, only a certain percentage of persons with that gene will actually present with Parkinson's. The rest complete their life span prior to developing symptoms of the disease (interview with Dr. Greene, 1996).

It has also been suggested that the toxin which causes dopamine producing cell death is something to which we are all exposed. Dr. Côté wonders if perhaps some people are more resistant to the effects of this toxin than others. Those who are not resistant develop PD. Other studies indicate that people with PD may not be able to remove the environmental toxins from their bodies as efficiently as others (Tanner et al., 1987).

One hypothesis is that there is something in rural environments which affects the development of PD. A Canadian researcher reported in 1993 that several studies he had conducted showed higher risk for PD among rural residents of Canada and lower "substantia nigra neuronal counts" in these areas (Rajput, 1993: 651). Two studies often compared to show the difference between PD rates by race also indicate the difference rates between city and rural environments. According to Schoenberg, a Baltimore study showed significantly higher rates of PD in whites than blacks (1987). It is implied that this study used doctors' records and could be influenced by the under-utilization of medical care by minority populations. His own door-to-door survey in Copiah County, Mississippi in a biracial community showed near equal levels of PD in white and black residents. Schoenberg's purpose is to show racial equity in the populations affected by this disease. Rajput, in his article, points out that the commonness of the environment in a door-to-door survey emphasizes the probability of an environmental factor (1993). The problem with this survey is that the investigators in the Copiah County study were looking for PD. They acknowledge 32 percent of the cases among whites and 58 percent among blacks were diagnosed at the time of the survey (Schoenberg, 1987). This creates suspicions about the accuracy of his case diagnoses. More importantly, focusing on race in comparing these two studies, clouds the difference in environments. The studies are depicting an urban environment versus a rural environment but neither article (Schoenberg or Rajput) discusses the effect of this difference.

Childhood environment is another consideration in the search for causes. Since this disease normally presents at least after age 40, and more likely after age 60, a slow acting agent has been suggested as the cause. According to this theory, exposure to the agent occurs early in life and damages the cells such that they degenerate more quickly. Another slow-acting theory is that constant low level exposure to a certain agent results over time in a buildup in the body which eventually causes PD (Tanner, 1990). Some studies have shown that in families with more than one sibling affected by PD the age at which the disease presented was related to the length of time they shared a common environment. The longer the environment was maintained, the earlier the disease appeared (Rajput, 1993).

Another possible explanation is an in-utero exposure that affects the brain as it is developing. Tipton suggests in his article that the effects of this exposure are only seen when the dopamine producing cells begin their natural deterioration process (1995). Another possibility is that the toxin's effects cause early death of some cells so that once the cells near the end of their natural life cycle, fewer cells remain than in non-PD affected people.

POSSIBLE ENVIRONMENTAL AGENTS

Some studies have identified possible agents that cause Parkinson-like symptoms and degeneration. The most famous is MPTP, which is a drug that was first produced by substance abusers attempting to make a narcotic. Several studies of people who experimented with this substance showed an instant development of some Parkinson-like symptoms but more importantly, autopsies indicated a similar pattern of neuron death and lewy bodies in the brain in MPTP victims and Parkinsonians (interview with Dr. Côté, 1996; interview with Dr. Greene, 1996; Tanner, 1990; Tanner et al., 1987). It is important to note that MPTP itself is not a toxic substance. When it is metabolized in the brain it creates a byproduct known as MPTP+ which does have toxic interactions with the cells in question (interview with Dr. Côté,

1996; interview with Dr. Greene, 1996; Tanner, 1990). Investigators believe that there may be naturally occurring environmental toxins which cause similar chemical reactions in the body as MPTP does, only over a longer period of time (Langston, 1987).

Several possible substances have been identified in rural communities in connection with the higher rates of disease found in these areas as mentioned earlier. One suspect is well water (Tipton, 1995; Tanner et al., 1987). Other studies based in Saskatchewan, Quebec, and Sweden identify higher concentrations of wood industries (paper mills, wood mills, saw mills) in areas where the incidence of PD was higher (Dr.Côté, 1996; Tanner, 1990; Tanner et al., 1987; Schoenberg, 1987). The Sweden study also indicated an increase of PD in areas with an emphasis on steel alloy and metal production (Tanner, 1990). Pesticide use has also been hypothetically linked to the development of PD (Schoenberg, 1987).

Manganese is another suspect substance. Manganese miners and others who work with manganese have been reported as showing Parkinson's symptoms (Schulte, 1996; interview with Dr. Côté, 1996; interview with Dr. Greene, 1996; Tipton, 1995). This has been associated with the formation of oxygen free-radicals which are thought to be key actors in the death of the cell mitochondria (Tipton, 1995). Iron is another potential toxin affecting the development of Parkinson's Disease. Higher levels of iron tend to be present in persons afflicted with neurodegenerative disorders. Some researchers believe that iron is responsible for the development of oxygen free-radicals; others wonder if higher iron production is "a response to neurodegeneration" (Tipton, 1995: 432).

The effect of industrialization on PD is unclear. While there is a higher rate in areas with certain types of production occurring, it seems that rural areas over all have higher rates of PD. The higher rates of the disease tend to be in countries with a longer history of industrialization as compared to newly modernized countries (Tipton, 1995). There also appear to be more cases of PD in the northern United States than the southern United States. Some would attribute this to industrial toxins (Tanner, 1990). The problem with an industrial explanation is that the disease has been identified since 1817 so at least some variation of the toxin would have to have been in the environment since the first days of industrialization. Also, this argument will be proven valid only if it can be shown that the disease did not exist prior to James Parkinson's discovery of it (Tanner, 1990). There is some argument that PD may have existed for centuries prior to its discovery. The discussion claims that because PD is the acquisition of several disparate symptoms, identification could not take place until a group of people with similar symptoms were living in close quarters (industrialization). They claim descriptions of people experiencing Parkinsonism exist in early literature (ed. "Discussion" 1990).

Another hypothetical cause of PD which is neither biological nor environmental is head trauma. This has been varyingly described as one which causes "an insult to the substantia nigra in early to mid-adult life" (Langston, 1987); one which was minor and caused little noticeable damage at the time (Tanner et al., 1987); a childhood injury (Tanner, 1990). Schoenberg found "head trauma [to be] positively associated with Parkinson's disease" (1987).

OTHER ISSUES

There has been a wide discussion of a supposedly protective effect of smoking cigarettes. It seems that smokers have a significantly lower incidence rate of PD (Tanner, 1990; Schoenberg, 1987). Some studies may have found a positive interaction of carbon monoxide with oxygen free-radicals that decreases the harm these free-radicals can cause (Tanner, 1990). However, several other studies have shown no real difference in rates of PD among smokers and non-smokers. Other studies have not been able to prove a dose-response effect exists for smoking and PD (Tanner, 1990). Tanner, Langston and Schoenberg in their various articles suggest that the explanation may be a "predisposition" among those who develop PD to dislike smoking. They report it is unclear if this is psychological or physiological; related to the disease or coincidental.

SUGGESTIONS FOR FURTHER RESEARCH

Finding a definitive causal agent for Parkinson's disease has been elusive. For over one hundred and seventy-five years, theories about the cause of idiopathic PD have gained and lost popularity but none have ever been proven. The balance usually swings between environmental and genetic causes. For now, at least, a viral cause has been ruled out. While arguments on either side of the issue remain strong, much is left unexplained. An example is Rochester, Minnesota. For close to 35 years, the incidence rates in Rochester have been constant at 16-21/100,000 per year (Tanner, 1987). This is the highest rate known in a nonindustrial area according to some morbidity surveys. Yet other studies have shown these numbers to be ambiguous. Either way, no one has as yet determined why the rate would be so high or so constant in this region, however, it would seem that an environmental explanation would be the most plausible.

The greatest difficulty in locating an environmental cause in a long onset disease is the forced reliance on patients' memories (Tanner, 1990). It will be particularly difficult for patients to recall exposure to items that seemed insignificant at the time if the disease does turn out to result from childhood exposure. The final complication in this investigation is that it seems much of the evidence can be used to support either theory. An example to think about: does the random familial pattern of the disease support the environmental cause theory because families have similar environments or the genetic predisposition theory because family members have common genes?

REFERENCES

Côté, Lucien J., MD. Neurological Institute, Columbia Presbyterian Medical Center. Interview, September 27, 1996.

Ed. "Discussion." *Neurology.* 40 (Suppl 3):30-31. October 1990.

Greene, Paul, MD. Neurological Institute, Columbia Presbyterian Medical Center. Personal Communication, October 7, 1996.

Hachinski, Vladmir, MD, DSc. "Parkinson's Disease: An Environmental Disease?" *Archives of Neurology.* 50:656. June 1993.

Langston, J. William. "MPTP: Insights into the Etiology of Parkinson's Disease." *European Neurology.* 26(Suppl 1): 2-10. 1987.

Lees, A.J., "Is deprenyl (selegiline) a safe treatment for Parkinson's Disease?" *British Medical Journal.* 311:1602-1607, 1995. Web Page.

Rajput, Ali H., MBBS, FRCPC. "Environmental Causation of Parkinson's Disease." *Archives of Neurology.* 50:651-652. June 1993.

Schoenberg, Bruce S. "Environmental risk factors for Parkinson's Disease: The epidemiologic evidence." *Canadian Journal of Neurological Sciences.* 14:407-413. 1987.

Schulte, Paul A., PhD, Burnett, Carol A., MS, Boeniger, Mark F., MS, Johnson, Jeffrey, PhD. "Neurodegenerative Disease: Occupational Occurrence and Potential Risk Factors, 1982-1991." *American Journal of Public Health.* 86(9):1281-1288. September 1996.

Tanner, Caroline M., MD, Langston, J. William, MD. "Do environmental toxins cause Parkinson's disease? A critical review." *Neurology.* 40 (Suppl 3):17-30. October 1990.

Tanner, Caroline M., MD, Chen, Biao, Wang, Wen-Zhi et al. "Environmental factors in the etiology of Parkinson's Disease." *Canadian Journal of Neurological Sciences.* 14:419-423. 1987.

The Sam and Rose Stein Institute for Research on Aging, University of California at San Diego School of Medicine. "UCSD Researchers Search for Understanding of Parkinson's Disease. Web Page. June 1995.

Tipton, K.F. "Might environmental factors contribute to neurodegenerative diseases?" *Biochemical Society Transactions.* 23(2):429-435. May 1995.

Oral Health, Dental Care
and Quality of Life Issues
in Parkinson's Disease

David Kaplan

Quality is defined by the *American Heritage Dictionary* (1978) in general terms, as "characteristic or attribute of something; a property; a feature" and in linguistics as "the character of a vowel sound determined by the size and shape of the oral cavity and the amount of resonance with which the sound is produced."

Quality of life, for people with Parkinson's disease (PD), may well be expressed in terms of the linguistic definition and its implications for daily living.

Dentistry and dental care speak uniquely to the quality of life in general, more specifically to the medically compromised, and especially to those with PD. The oral apparatus is singularly involved in nutrition, speech and, from birth, the psychological aspects of hunger, fear, and sensual expression. Diagnosing dental problems, correcting and maintaining this oral apparatus in PD patients is often hampered, if not totally frustrated, by the physical, psychological, and medical intervention sequelae of PD.

Given the scope of oral input to patient well-being, the dearth of pertinent current literature specifically on the dental care of PD persons leaves the practitioner with more questions than answers. For example, the Fourth Edition of *Dental Management of the Medically Compromised Patient* Little and Falace (1993), has no specific reference to PD care.

With our rapidly aging population it is surprising that epidemiologic litera-

David Kaplan, DDS, is Associate Professor of Dentistry (Ret.), School of Dental and Oral Surgery, Columbia University, New York, NY 10032.

[Haworth co-indexing entry note]: "Oral Health, Dental Care and Quality of Life Issues in Parkinson's Disease." Kaplan, David. Co-published simultaneously in *Loss, Grief & Care* (The Haworth Press, Inc.) Vol. 8, No. 3/4, 2000, pp. 87-92; and: *Parkinson's Disease and Quality of Life* (ed: Côté et al.) The Haworth Press, Inc., 2000, pp. 87-92. Single or multiple copies of this article are available for a fee from The Haworth Document Delivery Service [1-800-342-9678, 9:00 a.m. - 5:00 p.m. (EST). E-mail address: getinfo@haworthpressinc.com].

ture describing even the general oral health status of older adults in the U.S. is sparse. As of 1993, according to Douglass et al. (1993), there has been no community-based oral health survey on a representative sample of the 65-and-older population in an entire U.S. Public Health region.

The general age of PD patients places many of their ailments among those associated with the elderly. Therefore, their oral health problems come under the purview of geriatric dentistry although Allen (1990) states that there is some evidence that PD is found among younger adults as well.

Contrasted to the almost minuscule literature on the oral health and care of PD patients, geriatric dentistry enjoys voluminous references. It is logical, therefore, to consider the oral health quality of life of PD individuals primarily from a geriatric point of view with regard to stage of aging, symptoms, problems, drug reactions, etc., and then overlay this with the specific entities of PD with which they interact.

Looking at mental health in aging which directly affects the quality of life, "depression is the most frequently diagnosed of the three prevalent forms of late life psychopathosis, with secondary or reactive depression of major concern" (Papas 1991: 31). Parkinson's itself, or in combination with L-dopa among other drugs, may also produce depressive symptoms. If the dental team is to assist in improving the quality of life of PD individuals, the differential diagnosis and recognition of possible multiple inputs must be understood.

Pharmacologic side effects are of particular concern specifically where they affect the masticatory apparatus. A study of levodopa induced on-off motor fluctuations in PD as related to jaw movements by Karlsson et al. (1992) describes the increase in mandibular velocity and amplitude of movement following medication and also records a significant decreased occlusal level phase duration in the on state. This may account for the results, noted later, of decreasing the freeway space in denture construction.

"Phenytoin is known to induce gingival hyperplasia in the presence of poor oral hygiene" (Niessen and Jones 1987: 67), while anticholinergic regimens inhibit salivary gland function leading to xerostomia. Absent the antibacterial, lubricating, remineralizing, and buffering action of saliva, the patient is at increased risk of developing caries, periodontal disease and dysfunctions of speech, chewing, swallowing, and taste.

As PD progresses, autonomic dysfunction and mental symptoms increase and it becomes more difficult to reduce Parkinsonian symptoms without increasing these side effects. Impaired muscular and coordinative functions, added to the disadvantageous pharmacologic reactions, contribute heavily to the difficulties in maintaining oral hygiene.

Until 1992, no significant studies describing the oral status in PD patients compared with the situation in the general population of corresponding age had been done. The 1992 study found that the PD group had more teeth and less caries than a control group of corresponding age, but that salivary secretion rates were significantly lower with advancing PD symptoms. It was concluded that motor impairment and autonomic dysfunction adversely affect the oral health maintenance in PD persons relative to the degree of severity of the disease (Persson, Osterberg, Granerus, Karlsson 1992).

Flossing, brushing and rinsing functions are major components of oral hygiene and home care programs. These activities require muscle-eye coordination, digital dexterity and tongue-cheek-lip control. Tremor and the associated loss and/or lessening of the above faculties mitigate against effective oral hygiene procedures.

Understanding the reactions of the present drugs of choice in the specific individual is thus essential for the dental team. Field (1991) noted some positive results in delaying or stopping the development of PD with the use of Eldepryl.

A 1993 paper by Ishikawa and Miyatake reported the relief of tremor, rigidity, bradykinesia and gait disturbance in six early onset PD patients by smoking cigarettes. These effects lasted for 10 to 30 minutes, relieving the symptoms in the off-period and then disappeared rapidly. Smoking additional cigarettes did not produce alleviation of symptoms of the same magnitude. The report stated that nicotine has not been used clinically because of its harmful effects, but that it pointed the way toward new strategies for the treatment of PD.

Research in, and the development of, drugs better capable of easing oral therapeutic care, both for the patient and practitioner, should be the focus of a consortium of the Parkinson's Disease Foundation, the National Institute of Dental Research, and the American Association for Dental Research. Columbia University School of Dental and Oral Surgery would be an appropriate site for clinic evaluation.

Parenthetically, today's dental student, especially at Columbia, is far more medically oriented than in past generations. Physical diagnosis, hospital rounds and a multitude of ancillary courses relating to overall patient health make them more aware of pathologies that affect their dental services. However, PD has not been given the clinical exposure necessary for their familiarization with the special physical, and even more so psychologic, needs of these patients. Since PD patient are not generally seen in our clinics, it would be advantageous to dental students' education and their future patients' welfare for them to be invited on PD rounds wherever possible.

Patient care begins with diagnosis and Parkinson's has many dental, oral and maxillofacial manifestations each affecting patient management. Tremors may involve the head, neck, tongue, cheeks and mandible, making therapeutic treatment difficult, particularly when the patient's behavior changes from moment to moment (Jolly et al. 1989). Xerostomia can increase decay and decrease prosthetic function. Oral prostheses function optimally with healthy tissues upon which appliances can rest comfortably without causing irritation. Dry tissues produce denture sores. Speaking and masticatory functions are compromised as oral irritations develop, affecting nutrition. Loose dentures are socially embarrassing and further discomfort PD patients who struggle to overcome a tendency to withdraw. Uncontrolled facial muscles can dislodge maxillary dentures and an over-active tongue may displace and even eject a mandibular denture (Jolly, Paulson, Paulson and Pike 1989).

The PD patient requires the most careful history taking and clinical examination in light of the problems inherent in their physical and psychologic problems. Franks and Hedegard (1973: 52) note that the elderly in general have an intellectual rigidity presenting difficulty in adapting from one task to another often resulting in slower performance and in becoming pedantic in their responses. This will further complicate the history-taking and the examination process but must be pursued with far more sophistication and insight than is normally required.

Treatment planning must take into account the patient's ability to perform, or have performed by others, the oral hygiene procedures necessary for the maintenance of the natural dentition and/or appliances. Cosmetic needs, treatment phobias, psychosocial and behavioral aspects of past history call for comprehensive team analysis to develop the optimal approach to treatment.

The primary care physician, neurologist, social worker, nutritionist, psychologist, personal care aide and spouse can have positive input from the best time of day for the dental appointment to the choice of pharmacologic approach.

The therapeutic goal is to restore the dentition to health, comfort and function, thus improving the quality of life following delivery of care. There is, however, the need to improve the quality of life during treatment. Cooperation, even if only able to be given on a minimal basis, and a sense of ease while under treatment, makes further care more easily accepted and more easily rendered. The guidelines are simple: gentleness, a caring attitude, a quiet atmosphere and an understanding of the patient's limitations. Consultation with the patient's physician is most helpful–to both health providers.

Suggestions for improving the quality of life during dental treatment of PD patients come from many other service specialties. An ophthalmologist, Dr. Kenneth Barasch, questioned about PD patient clinical care, told me that they are generally very light-sensitive and close their eyes when approached by an examiner. They then respond to directions such as "Open your eyes" by shutting them tightly. He attributes the latter actions to a garbling in the cerebral ganglia and suggests that verbal directions not be given, rather, place the head in the desired position and open the eyes manually, which the patient readily accepts.

The parallels to dentistry are clear–provide the patient with disposable plastic sunshades, approach slowly and manually position the head and mandible gently but without verbal direction.

Audiologists may have other insights. A hygienist noted frequent cheek biting and a British dentist (Hussein 1989) developed a gum shield to protect the cheeks and tongue from that source of trauma.

Speech therapists are helpful in modifying prosthesis design to improve phonetics. This may sometimes conflict with the prosthodontist's technique of reducing interocclusal distance to favor ridge preservation and lessen masticatory pressure, but here is where a team approach not only avoids single provider tunnel vision, but also works to the ultimate improvement of the patient's overall comfort and function.

A multidisciplinary effort encompassing the total dental care needs of PD people could bring together the basic science, clinical knowledge and psychosocial insight needed for comprehensive oral health care. The indications are clear and the means available.

REFERENCES

Allen, W.A. 1990. "New Studies on Parkinson's Disease Drug." *British Dental Journal*, 22(6): 150 (letter).

American Heritage Dictionary, New College Edition, 1978. Houghton Mifflin, Boston.

Barasch, Kenneth, Personal Communication.

Douglass, C.W., A.M. Jette, C.H. Fox, S.L. Tennstedt, A. Joshi, H.A. Feldman, S.M. McGuire, and J.B. McKinlay. 1993. "Oral Health Status of the Elderly in New England." *Journal of Gerontology: Medical Sciences*, 48(2): M39-M46.

Field, R. 1991. "Dr. Parkinson's Cruel Disease." American Health, 10(7):55-58.

Franks, A.S.T, and B. Hedegard 1973. Aging and Oral Health, Blackwell Scientific, Oxford.

Hussein, S.B. 1989. "Use of a Gum Shield for Parkinson's Disease Patients." *British Dental Journal*, 166(9): 320 (letter).

Ishikawa, A. and T. Miyatake. 1993. "Effects of Smoking in Patients with Early-onset Parkinson's Disease." *Journal of the Neurological Sciences*, 117(1-2): 28-32.

Jolly, D.E., R.B. Paulson and G.W. Paulson. 1989. "Parkinson's Disease: A Review and Recommendations for Dental Management." *Special Care in Dentistry*, 9(3): 74-78.

Karlsson, S., M. Persson and B. Johnels. 1992. "Levodopa Induced ON-OFF Motor Fluctuations in Parkinson's Disease Related to Rhythmical Masticatory Jaw Movements." *Journal of Neurology, Neurosurgery and Psychiatry*, 55: 304-307.

Little, J.A., and D.A. Falace 1993. *Dental Management of the Medically Compromised Patient*, 4th Edition. Mosby, St. Louis.

Niessen, L.C. and J.A. Jones. 1987. Professional Care for Patients with Dementia."
    Gerontology, 6(2): 67-71.
Papas, A.S. 1991 "Aging and Oral Health." In *Geriatric Dentistry, Psychologic Aspects of Aging*, St. Louis: Mosby pp. 31-34.
Persson, M., T. Osterberg, A-K Granerus and S. Karlsson. 1992. "Influence of Parkinson's Disease on Oral Health." *Acta Odontologica Scandinavia*, 50(1):37-42.

RECOMMENDED READING

Iacopino, A.M. and W.F. Wathen. 1993. "Geriatric Prosthodontics: An Overview, Part 1. Pretreatment Considerations." *Quintessence International*, 24(4).
Tryon, A.F., 1986. *Oral Health and Aging*. Littleton, Massachusetts: PSG Publishing Co.

Managing Incontinence
in People with Parkinson's Disease

Steven A. Kaplan
Ben Z. Jacobs

One of our jobs as neuro-urologists, is to treat urologic problems related to neurologic disease and one of the most devastating complications of Parkinson's disease is urinary incontinence. It really is one of the most devastating problems, in fact, that any person can have. It impacts on patients' independence and their self-esteem. In fact, incontinence is probably the last great untreated condition in this country today. It's been estimated that 20 to 25 million Americans have urinary incontinence. That's more than the combined number of patients with diabetes and heart disease together. How is incontinence managed? The simple solution is for the patient to wear diapers. That is the level of sophistication for most patients, and unfortunately, it is the level of sophistication of most physicians and other health care providers. What can be done? People can be educated that there are a host of options and in fact, for the most part, urinary incontinence is a treatable condition. It is not necessarily curable, but it is certainly treatable.

What is urinary incontinence, in terms of definition? It is the involuntary loss of urine per the urethra or the urinary channel that is sufficient to be a problem. The key word, particularly for patients with PD, is involuntary. Different people have varying thresholds of what bothers them. There are people who are devastated by a couple of drops and there are people who are very, very wet but become accustomed to it. The input of the patient is very important and dramatic.

Steven A. Kaplan, MD, is Herbert H. Irving Assistant Professor of Urology and Director, Neurourology and Prostate Center, College of Physicians and Surgeons, Columbia University, New York, NY 10032.

[Haworth co-indexing entry note]: "Managing Incontinence in People with Parkinson's Disease." Kaplan, Steven A., and Ben Z. Jacobs. Co-published simultaneously in Loss, Grief & Care (The Haworth Press, Inc.) Vol. 8, No. 3/4, 2000, pp. 93-97; and: Parkinson's Disease and Quality of Life (ed: Côté et al.) The Haworth Press, Inc., 2000, pp. 93-97. Single or multiple copies of this article are available for a fee from The Haworth Document Delivery Service [1-800-342-9678, 9:00 a.m. - 5:00 p.m. (EST). E-mail address: getinfo@haworthpressinc.com].

Briefly, in terms of the innervation of the urinary bladder, most of the innervation of the bladder is cholinergic and therefore medical therapy is geared to that level. When prostate disease is treated, the anti-cholinergic types of medications are what is important and for the majority of Parkinson's patients, these are the types of medications that we have to consider. The major reason why patients with PD have disease of their bladder is this: they lack the normal inhibition of bladder contractions. In effect, most patients with Parkinson's disease who have urinary problems, have over-activity of their bladder. These patients have increased urge to void and urge incontinence. The reason is they have lost the inhibitory capacity in the brain. In terms of the mechanism of urinary incontinence, it is sort of common sense. Basically, as I explain to my patients, it is similar to the relationship between a faucet and a sink. That is, when the pressure of the faucet is higher than the pressure of the sink, or the resistance of the sink, there is going to be leakage. The same thing is true when the pressure of the bladder is greater than what the outlet or sphincter mechanism can give, there will be leakage. It is very important for us to clinically categorize patients appropriately in terms of their level of incontinence.

For the most part patients with Parkinson's have what we call detrusor over-activity. That is the detrusor or bladder muscle contracts when it should not. Patients have an urge to go, can not control it and wet themselves on the way to the bathroom. That is the problem for the vast majority of patients in terms of the etiology of incontinence. There is also what we call stress incontinence. This refers to physical stress. This is commonly found in women; classically, it is the woman who has had a number of children and her bladder has dropped down a little bit, therefore the sphincter mechanism does not work. What makes bladder dysfunction in PD patients very difficult and different than any other type of neuro-urologic condition, different than patients with strokes or brain tumors, is the fact that they have an over-activity of their bladder muscle associated with weakness of the muscle. In other words, there can be detrusor under-activity in a sense with detrusor over-activity. A person experiences too many contractions but they are not strong. This could be considered weak over-activity. This happens about 30 to 40 percent of the time in patients with Parkinson's disease. This is important because medications or treatments that are geared toward slowing the bladder down, may slow it too much and because the bladder is inherently weak, the patients may not be able to void very well. This is one dilemma in treating Parkinson's patients with incontinence.

The most common test that we do is urodynamic testing. The purpose of urodynamic testing is two-fold. We aim to reproduce the patient's symptoms in a controlled environment but more importantly to identify those risk factors which will ultimately hurt or affect the demise of that patient. Most patients obviously will not die of incontinence but they can die from some of the repercussions of the underlying mechanisms of their incontinence. Those that we worry about include dyssynergia or high pressure in the bladder, poor compliance or loss of bladder elasticity, vesico-ureteral reflux or urinary contents backing up into the kidney and finally, probably the worse thing, an indwelling catheter. Any of these four problems may ultimately lead to kidney dysfunction. It is interesting, although not necessarily part of the topic, that soldiers during World War II and the Korean War who had spinal cord injury, died not because of their spinal cord injury but because of renal failure. The reason for this is that we did not know how to manage their urologic dysfunction and certainly these are the risk factors we want to avoid. We have mentioned the different types of urinary incontinence and again, just to review, for the most part, patients with Parkinson's will have urge incontinence. Functional incontinence is also an important part because many patients with PD can not run to the bathroom. So, they may have the urge and recognize it and want to control it, but because of the bradykinesia and various other problems with mobility they can not get to the bathroom in time. This problem can be managed with just changing the environment of that patient, that is bringing the bathroom to the patient, rather than the patient going to the bathroom.

In Parkinson's disease particularly, the most common urodynamic findings that we see are what we call detrusor hyperreflexia or over-activity of the bladder. There is also a phenomenon of delay in the relaxation of the sphincter, or dyssynergia. Normally, when a person wants to void, the sphincter relaxes, the bladder contracts and the urine flows. Unfortunately, there are patients with Parkinson's who have a delay of this relaxation and therefore they are urinating against an obstruction. That is, they are urinating against their sphincter and that can cause problems. In addition, some patients as I mentioned before, not only have over-activity of their bladder, it is weakly over-active. So they have what we call impaired bladder contractility. Something else that is very common as men get older and afflicts men with PD as well, is benign prostate hyperplasia or BPH. Physicians can not just take care of the Parkinson's disease part of the bladder, they have to take care of the prostate which also tends to complicate things.

To briefly discuss some of the therapies available to treat PD patients, We will begin with the treatment of dyssynergia. This can be treated, interestingly enough, with a technique that we have used frequently at Columbia-Presbyterian, and that is biofeedback. This trains the patient to relax the sphincter muscle during voiding and thus lower the bladder pressure. Biofeedback has been very effective for some patients with this type of problem. The major category of therapy we use in addition to biofeedback is pharmacologic. The most common medications are the class that we call anticholinergics and that is because, as I alluded to earlier, most of the innervation to the bladder is cholinergic or parasympathetic to be more precise. Some drugs work at the receptor site, and these are the most commonly used agents. An example of this class is Propanthalene, or Probanthine. Other agents may induce intracellular blockade, such as oxybutinin or Ditropan, and Levsinex. It is important to consider that when the bladder is slowed down, the patient is put at risk of retention because that patient may not have strong enough bladder contractions to urinate. One other point to bear in mind is, as I mentioned before, the coexistence of neurogenic bladder dysfunction and BPH in men. Men with Parkinson's disease are often in the same age group as men at risk for an enlarged prostate, and there are particular risk factors to contemplate. One prognostic indicator of potentially favorable outcome is the presence of primarily obstructive voiding symptoms such as diminished urinary stream and straining to void. Those patients with relatively large bladder capacities and good control of their sphincter, with mostly obstructive symptoms are likely to do well after therapeutic intervention for their BPH. Unfortunately, the majority of patients with Parkinson's disease who have BPH, complain of urge related symptoms such as frequency, urgency, urge incontinence and nocturia. When these patients are studied urodynamically, they are found to have involuntary bladder contractions, small bladder capacities with small residual volumes and absent or weak sphincter control. These are particularly difficult patients to manage because treatment of their BPH alone often fails to improve their voiding symptoms.

In the female patient with Parkinson's disease, the most common neuro-urologic condition affecting their bladder is, once again, involuntary contractions of their bladder. Patients can also have stress incontinence related to bladder prolapse, causing the loss of urine with coughing or sneezing. Our approach to the patient with pure urge incontinence involves both biofeedback and anti-cholinergic medication. Patients with mixed, or both urge and stress, incontinence will often show dramatic improvement with this approach as well. We try to avoid surgical correction of stress incontinence associated with bladder prolapse in these patients. They just do not do very well. One additional class of therapy is injectable collagen. Collagen injections have been used in cosmetic applications and we are now performing the procedure in the urinary channel. The collagen is injected via the cystoscope into the submucosal space of the urethra at the level of the bladder neck with a net bulking effect of the sphincter mechanism. Suitable candidates for this procedure are those with sphincteric incontinence with low leak point pressure. In women, this may be associated with the aging process. In men, sphincteric incontinence is most often found following prostate surgery.

There are additional types of treatment available to the PD patient with neurogenic bladder dysfunction, but the key message is that (1) it is something that a patient does not have to ignore; (2) it is not something that you have to live with. Diapers are not the best cure for incontinence–it is not appropriate for most patients. Most patients can be treated once the diagnosis is made and I would encourage PD patients and their health care providers to seek proper diagnosis and therapy.

Nursing Home Care as an Option

Bobba Jean Moody

For many people, the thought of going into a nursing home or arranging for a relative or loved one to be admitted to a nursing home is fraught with fear about how that person will respond and a general sense that the elderly or disabled are warehoused. This implies that in the worst case scenario the person is just thrown into a room, never taken out of bed, given poor nutrition, isolated, abandoned, and left to waste away alone. Families often think of nursing homes this way, as do patients, and families have promised their loved ones that they will never put them in this kind of environment.

In today's more sophisticated and knowledgeable society, warehousing has been greatly diminished. The consumers' advocates movement of the late 60's and 70's aggressively pushed for improvements in nursing home care. In New York State particularly, the New York State Department of Health and the accrediting bodies for nursing homes have demanded that consumers, patients, and families, have their rights respected and that they be treated well in any residential health care facility.

There are some wonderful nursing homes that provide a chockfull busy schedule morning to night with a good level of activity and entertainment. There are other people for residents to talk to, and there is space for time alone for individuals who need this. Now that the State monitors and regulates nursing homes, they have become more responsive to patients' needs. There is, in fact, a Patient Bill of Rights.

But how does one come to the conclusion that a relative or loved one needs to be in a nursing home? There are entitlement programs, the resources available in each community, home care; but for some people these no longer

Bobba Jean Moody, MSW, CSW, is Assistant Clinical Professor of Psychiatric Social Work, College of Physicians and Surgeons, Columbia University, New York, NY 10032.

[Haworth co-indexing entry note]: "Nursing Home Care as an Option." Moody, Bobba Jean. Co-published simultaneously in *Loss, Grief & Care* (The Haworth Press, Inc.) Vol. 8, No. 3/4, 2000, pp. 99-102; and: *Parkinson's Disease and Quality of Life* (ed: Côté et al.) The Haworth Press, Inc., 2000, pp. 99-102. Single or multiple copies of this article are available for a fee from The Haworth Document Delivery Service [1-800-342-9678, 9:00 a.m. - 5:00 p.m. (EST). E-mail address: getinfo@haworthpressinc.com].

work. They have reached the stage at which they are too debilitated or ill to be adequately cared for at home, and they need 24-hour care and supervision, and security that a nursing home can provide. When this time comes, the patients need a level of skilled care that most families are not able to provide, financially or otherwise. For some people who are still living at home, nursing home care is not the last resort, it is the first choice. These are people who feel isolated in their own home and cannot go out on their own. These individuals are frightened and confused, lonely, unable to get dressed, and cannot independently care for themselves. For them the idea of being with other people in a communal environment where they can socialize and be with others outweighs whatever advantage there is to staying at home. It is usually not thought of in these terms, but there are people who choose to go into a nursing home.

It is very hard for a family to think about placing a loved one in a nursing home, and this is one of the hardest aspects of being a caregiver. There are a number of factors that the family or other responsible individual needs to examine if placement in a facility is being considered.

EMOTIONAL FACTORS

Some patients feel responsible for the disruption their care causes in the family support system. They are pained by the sacrifices other family members have to make, such as giving up work, not being able to go out with friends, having to stay at home. In such situations, the patients themselves choose to go into a residential facility, feeling that they want to unburden their families. Think about how many daughters have had to give up their jobs when they have had to stay with their mother or father full time. Statistically, the most common situation is that of daughters taking care of mothers. This can destroy other family relationships, and parents may conclude that the sacrifices are too great and that it would be better to go into a nursing home than to disrupt their own family's lives. This then allows family reintegration and a more normal lifestyle. This situation is particularly true for "sandwich generation" families, those who are being squeezed between caring for their own children and for elderly parents at the same time. And it is the unusual family these days that has extended family members sufficient in number available to help out with the task.

This is an issue one might want to think about. What would life be like if one had the responsibility of caring for a relative full-time? What impact would it have on that life if you were to care for a mother or father, or spouse? Would one have to give up his/her job? How would it change your relationship with your spouse? With one's children? Would staying home all the time be difficult? Could one go out with friends? These are some of the things that parents think about when their children are their caregivers. In many cases, they make the decision that they do not want to disrupt their family's life and they want the family to have a more normal life.

As a caregiver, what personal unresolved issues would one have that would get played out and how stressful would that be? Would the stress destroy other relationships in one's life? With a husband or children? What about other brothers and sisters who do not help out? This is a very tense, highly emotionally charged time, when one becomes the caregiver for his/her relative. In the natural course of life, we all have very complicated feelings about those we are close to, especially our parents. We have a lot of positive feelings and a lot of negative ones, and the caregiver situation is set up to mobilize a whole confluence of feelings with marked intensity. These are difficult to deal with, especially on a daily, day-in, day-out basis–with no relief. It is also difficult to watch the ill person who has been the strong one becoming the weak one.

There are situations in which the relative or loved one becomes so debilitated that he/she cannot be managed in the home emotionally or physically. The emotional demands of taking care of someone with advanced Parkinson's disease are extremely stressful. There are relatives and loved ones of patients who cannot tolerate the pain that comes along with witnessing the increased debilitation and progression of this illness. They cannot tolerate the painful feelings that are evoked and triggered.

ANOTHER SIGNIFICANT FACTOR IS FINANCIAL

Most of us do not have either the insurance coverage or the personal finances to be able to maintain the patient at home, even if that is where the loved one wants to be. The patient often needs 12 to 24 hours of assistance in the home. Financial assistance for care is limited. Medicare is not designed for funding long-term care for illness but for acute illness, and it is the unusual family member who is able to sustain a totally debilitated relative in the home.

CHOOSING A NURSING HOME

It can be reassuring to families and patients to know that nursing homes are regulated and there are agencies available to protect the patient. In addition, there is usually a social worker at the nursing home available to help residents adjust to the environment. Social workers also help with the transitions from a level of independent functioning to more dependence on others, help with problem situations, and assist with transfers when the situation does not work out. F.R.I.A., The Friends and Relatives of Institutionalized Aged, provides a number of resources for help in choosing a nursing home and in monitoring nursing homes. The New York City Department of Aging, Division of Residential and Nursing Home Affairs, also offers help and guidance in this area. Judith Brickman has suggested that at least four or five places be visited and that for the first visit one should never go alone.

When considering a nursing home there are some critical things to think about. Among them are:

1. Location–so friends and relatives can visit.
2. Staff ratio within the different disciplines.
3. Availability of physician consultation routinely, and for medical emergencies.
4. Quality of food.
5. Types, frequency, and availability of activities and recreation. (Some even have barbers and hairdressers on site.)
6. Inclusion of physical therapy and occupational therapy in activities.

CONCLUSION

In conclusion, nursing homes should not be thought of necessarily as a choice of last resort, and for some individuals the nursing home is overall the best environment. The family can feel that patient is being taken care of, and the patient can feel relief from burdening the caregiver. However, the family needs to be involved in choosing and visiting nursing homes so they can make an informed decision. Residence in a nursing home can be seen as a potential opportunity and is, in fact, a viable option for many patients and family members.

Health Care Proxies

Walter I. Nathan

INTRODUCTION

A Health Care Proxy [sometimes referred to as a HCP] is a written instrument which permits the principal to designate an agent [sometimes referred to as a Health Care Agent or HCA] to make health care decisions when the principal is not competent to do so. Health Care Proxies are authorized by Article 29-C of the New York Public Health Law.[1] A *health care decision* is any decision to consent to or refuse to consent to health care, e.g., whether to have an operation, whether to administer particular medications, or any medications, whether to have the principal placed on a respirator, whether to have blood transfusions.[2] A HCA also has the power to direct that treatment previously undertaken be withdrawn.[3] A HCA will not have the authority to make decisions concerning artificial hydration or artificial nutrition unless that authority is specifically expressed in the Health Care Proxy.[4] A HCA does not have the authority to direct a health care provider to take affirmative steps to end the principal's life, e.g., a HCA may direct that the principal be taken off a respirator, but a HCA can not authorize a health care provider to inject the principal with a drug which will cause respiration to stop.[5] A HCA may receive [what would otherwise be] confidential medical information necessary to make informed decisions regarding the principal's health care.[6]

THE PRINCIPAL

Any "competent adult"[7] may execute a HCP as principal. The law provides a broad presumption of competency.[8] Physical disability is not a bar to execution of a HCP.[9]

Walter I. Nathan, Esquire, is an Attorney at Law, New York, NY.

[Haworth co-indexing entry note]: "Health Care Proxies." Nathan, Walter I. Co-published simultaneously in *Loss, Grief & Care* (The Haworth Press, Inc.) Vol. 8, No. 3/4, 2000, pp. 103-109; and: *Parkinson's Disease and Quality of Life* (ed: Côté et al.) The Haworth Press, Inc., 2000, pp. 103-109. Single or multiple copies of this article are available for a fee from The Haworth Document Delivery Service [1-800-342-9678, 9:00 a.m. - 5:00 p.m. (EST). E-mail address: getinfo@haworthpressinc.com].

THE HEALTH CARE AGENT

Any adult may be named as a HCA. The nomination must be of a specific individual, not by title or description [e.g., Jane Doe, but not the Minister of The Green Lane Church], not a corporation or professional corporation. There are limitations and restrictions on treating physicians, and operators, administrators, etc., of a "facility" where the principal is a patient acting as Health Care Agents, except for relatives.[10] A logical choice for a Health Care Agent would be a close relative or friend. The HCA's situation may be complicated and the HCA's decisions may be subject to special scrutiny if the HCA is or might be a beneficiary of the principal's estate. There is no authority for "joint" Health Care Agents but the principal may name an individual as alternate Health Care Agent in the Health Care Proxy.[11] Divorce revokes the appointment of a Health Care Agent.[12]

THE HEALTH CARE AGENT'S DUTIES

After consultation with a licensed physician, registered nurse, licensed clinical psychologist or certified social worker, the HCA shall make health care decisions (a) in accordance with the principal's wishes, including the principal's religious and moral beliefs, or (b) if the principal's wishes are not known and cannot reasonably be determined, in accordance with the principal's best interests, but the HCA has no authority to make decisions concerning artificial nutrition and hydration unless the principal's wishes in that regard can be determined.[13] Therefore, if the HCA is to have authority to make decisions concerning artificial nutrition or hydration, that authority must be expressly stated in the Health Care Proxy.

OBLIGATIONS OF HEALTH CARE PROVIDERS

If the patient submits a Health Care Proxy to a health care provider, the health care provider has an obligation to include the Health Care Proxy [or copy of the Health Care Proxy] in the principal's medical record.[14] A health care provider shall comply with health care decisions made by a HCA in good faith under a Health Care Proxy as if such decisions had been made by the principal.[15]

A health care provider or family member or friend may bring a judicial proceeding to determine the validity of a Health Care Proxy, or to remove a Health Care Agent who is not acting or who is acting in bad faith, or to override a decision made by a Health Care Agent who is acting in bad faith or has given instructions not in accord with the principal's wishes.[16]

WHEN THE HEALTH CARE AGENT CAN ACT

A HCA can act when a determination has been made that the principal lacks capacity to make health care decisions,[17] subject to overriding command by the principal,[18] unless a judicial determination is made that the principal lacks capacity to make health care decisions. The HCA's authority ends when the principal regains capacity.[19]

THE DETERMINATION THAT THE PRINCIPAL LACKS CAPACITY TO MAKE HEALTH CARE DECISIONS

A determination that the principal lacks capacity to make health care decisions shall be made by the attending physician to a reasonable degree of medical certainty. The determination shall be in writing and included in the patient's medical record, and shall contain a statement as to the cause and nature of the incapacity and the extent and probable duration. An attending physician must make continued written determinations of incapacity.[20] Decisions as to incapacity which may involve withdrawal or withholding of life sustaining treatment require that the attending physician consult with another physician.[21]

A HCA may request that an attending physician make a determination regarding capacity.

NOTICE OF THE DETERMINATION OF INCAPACITY

Notice of the determination that the principal lacks capacity to make health care decisions shall be given to the principal orally and in writing where there is any indication of the principal's ability to comprehend such notice. Notice must also be given to the Health Care Agent.[22]

PROTECTIONS FOR THE PRINCIPAL [PATIENT]

The HCA has no authority to act until the attending physician determines that the principal lacks capacity to make health care decisions.[23]

The principal must be notified of the determination of incapacity to make health care decisions.[24]

Notwithstanding a physician's determination that the principal lacks capacity to make health care decisions, if the principal objects to either the determination of incapacity or a health care decision by the HCA, the principal's objection or decision shall prevail unless a court of competent jurisdiction determines that the principal does not have capacity to make health care decisions.[25]

The attending physician must reconfirm the principal's lack of capacity to make health care decisions before complying with subsequent directives of the HCA.[26]

The HCA's authority terminates [subject to revival in the event of a later incapacity] if the attending physician determines that the principal has regained the capacity to make health care decisions.

The principal may provide that the Health Care Proxy expire on a particular date or on the occurrence of a specified event.[27]

A health care provider, family member, or close friend may bring a judicial proceeding to determine the validity of a Health Care Proxy, i.e., whether it was signed by the principal, whether it was properly witnessed, whether the principal was competent to execute the instrument, whether the execution of the instrument was procured through fraud or undue influence.

FORM OF THE HEALTH CARE PROXY

The law provides a sample form of Health Care Proxy.[28] However no particular format is required. The Health Care Proxy should be in writing and signed by the principal in the presence of two witnesses who should sign their names and addresses. I suggest that the Health Care Proxy be signed in a doctor's or lawyer's office in the expectation that the professional will document the execution and assist in establishing the *bona fides* of the instrument if it is challenged. The Health Care Proxy may contain "living will" instructions. The Health Care Proxy can not be executed on or as part of another form which includes a [non-health care] power of attorney.[29]

A sample Health Care Proxy is included at the end of this memorandum.

REVOCATION OF A HEALTH CARE PROXY

A Health Care Proxy may be revoked, orally or in writing, by notice to the HCA or to a health care provider[30] or by execution of a subsequent Health Care Proxy.[31] Unless otherwise specified, a Health Care Proxy is revoked by divorce.[32]

FORMS AND ADDITIONAL INFORMATION

The New York State Department of Health, Box 2000, Albany, NY 12220 will provide forms of Health Care Proxies and information about the law.

HEALTH CARE PROXY

I, Peter Patient, hereby appoint my sister, Ann Agent of 123 East 45th Street, New York, NY 10067 [212/999-XXXX], as my Health Care Agent to make any and all health care decisions for me, except to the extent that I state otherwise.

This Health Care Proxy shall take effect in the event I become unable to make my own health care decisions.

I do not want the process of my dying to be prolonged unless that is the unintended consequence of efforts made with a reasonable prospect that if successful they will restore me to a cognitive and conscious state. If I suffer from an injury, disease, illness or other physical or mental condition which renders me unable to make medical decisions on my own behalf, or leaves me unable to communicate with others meaningfully, and from which there is no reasonable prospect of recovery to a cognitive and conscious state, I direct that no medical treatments or procedures be used in my care or, if begun that such procedures [including without limitation: life support systems; intravenous or naso-gastric feeding, or other artificial nutrition; and, ventilation or respiration assistance] be discontinued, except to the extent necessary for my comfort or to alleviate pain. I specifically authorize my Health Care Agent to make decisions about artificial nutrition and hydration.

I direct my agent to make health care decisions in accordance with my wishes and instructions as stated above or as otherwise known to her. I also direct my agent to abide by any limitations on her authority as stated above or as otherwise known to her.

In the event Ann Agent is unable, unwilling, or unavailable to act as my Health Care Agent, I hereby appoint my cousin Alice Alternate of 99 Prospect Park West, Brooklyn, NY 11200 [718/111-ZZZZ] as my Health Care Agent.

I understand that, unless I revoke it, this proxy will remain in effect indefinitely.

    Signature:
      Address: 630 East 69th Street, New York, NY 10021
        Date: October ____, 1994

I declare that the person who signed this document is personally known to me and appears to be of sound mind and acting willingly and free from duress. He signed this document in my presence. I am not the person appointed as agent by this document.

Witness: Witness:
Address: Address:

NOTES

1. Unless otherwise indicated, references are to sections of the New York Public Health Law.

2. §2980 subd. 6

3. Examples of tragic situations resulting from the absence of a Health Care Proxy are *Westchester County Medical Center (O'Connor) v. Hall*, 534 NYS 2d 886 [Court of Appeals, 1988] and *Elbaum v. Grace Plaza of Great Neck*, 544 NYS 2d 840 [Second Dept, 1989]. In *Westchester County Medical Center*, the Court of Appeals ordered insertion of a naso-gastric feeding tube in a patient who had sustained substantial irreversible brain damage, was substantially paralyzed, severely demented, and profoundly incapacitated with no gag reflex, notwithstanding the opposition of family and testimony that the patient had declared that she would not want to be so treated. The Court of Appeals stated that as a condition of withholding treatment, there must be clear and convincing evidence that the patient held a firm and settled commitment to termination of life support under circumstances like those presented. In *Elbaum* the patient, who was in an irreversible, persistent vegetative state, had been distressed at her mother having been maintained by a naso-gastric feeding tube and asked her husband, children, and siblings to pledge that they would never permit her to be so maintained. A hearing **and an appeal** were required before the family was able to arrange for removal of a gastrointestinal feeding tube over opposition from the nursing home where the patient was being maintained. More than a year and a half elapsed between the time the family requested the nursing home to discontinue "feeding" through the gastric feeding tube and the appellate decision granting permission to do so.

4. §2982 subd. 2 (b)

5. The law establishing Health Care Proxies includes a Statement of Legislative intent which provides, in part, "(T)he legislature does not intend to authorize an agent to deny to the patient services that every patient would generally receive, such as appropriate food, water . . . ," and "This legislation confers no new rights regarding the provision or rejection of any specific health care treatment and affirms existing laws and policies which limit individual conduct, including those laws and policies against homicide, suicide, assisted suicide and mercy killing."

6. §2982 subd. 3

7. A person over the age of 18 years, or who is a parent, or who is married. §2980 subd. 1.

8. §2981 subd. 1.

9. §2982 subd. 2 (a)

10. §2981 subd. 6

11. §2981 subd. 6

12. §2985 subd. 1 (e)

13. §2982 subd. 2

14. §2984 subd. 1.

15. §2984 subd. 2

16. §2992

17. §2981 subd. 4 and §2983

18. §2983 subd. 5

19. §2983 subd. 7
20. 2983 subd. 6
21. §2983 subd. 1 (a)
22. §2983 subd. 3
23. §2983 subd. 1 (a)
24. §2983 subd. 3
25. §2983 subd. 5
26. §2983 subd. 6 (a)
27. §2981 subd. 5 (c)
28. §2981 subd. 5 (d)
29. §2981 subd. 5 (e)
30. §2985 subd. 1 (a)
31. §2985. subd 1 (b)
32. §2985 subd. 1 (e)

Fetal Tissue Implantation

D. Eugene Redmond, Jr.

Fetal Tissue Implantation has been responsible for an enormous amount of public interest and misinformation, and possibly, but hopefully not, misplaced hopes. One day that enthusiasm may be repaid. The neurotransplant program at Yale has been going on for a number of years and consists of two components: one, a program involving nonhuman primates using the MPTP model, and, second, the clinical studies at Yale with patients with Parkinson's disease. The rationale for the neural transplant operation comes from the understanding that many of the symptoms of Parkinson's Disease result from the loss of dopamine neurons in certain areas of the brain. The loss of these neurons has a number of effects, the most significant of which is impairment of the circuits involved with motor movement. The most dramatic effect of anything so far discovered useful for Parkinson's disease is that of dopamine agonist therapy and L-Dopa both of which essentially restore the function of these circuits by replacement. These drugs work very well for some patients, but in many patients have serious side effects and/or stop working after a period of time.

The idea behind transplantation is to take those missing dopamine neurons from some other source and implant them in the target area so that they can

D. Eugene Redmond, Jr., MD, is Professor of Psychiatry (in Surgery); Director of Yale Neural Transplant Program (Neurobehavior Laboratory), Yale University School of Medicine, New Haven, CT.

These studies were carried out by and in collaboration with J. R. Sladek, Jr., R. H. Roth, J. D. Elsworth, J. R. Taylor, T. J. Collier, D. D. Spencer, F. Naftolin, R. J. Robbins, K. L. Marek, T. Vollmer, C. Leranth, A. Gjedde, K. J. Sass, B. S. Bunney, P. Hoffer, L. H. Price, L. E. Kier, B. I. Gulanski, and C. Serrano. Studies were supported by NS24032, the Axion Research Foundation, the G. Harold and Leila Y. Mathers Foundation, other private donors, and Research Scientist Award MHOO643 to DER.

[Haworth co-indexing entry note]: "Fetal Tissue Implantation." Redmond, D. Eugene, Jr. Co-published simultaneously in *Loss, Grief & Care* (The Haworth Press, Inc.) Vol. 8, No. 3/4, 2000, pp. 111-114; and: *Parkinson's Disease and Quality of Life* (ed: Côté et al.) The Haworth Press, Inc., 2000, pp. 111-114. Single or multiple copies of this article are available for a fee from The Haworth Document Delivery Service [1-800-342-9678, 9:00 a.m. - 5:00 p.m. (EST). E-mail address: getinfo@haworthpressinc.com].

produce dopamine and replace the neurotransmitter. In the case of fetal tissue transplantation, these source cells would be dopamine neuroblasts–dopamine neuron precursor cells. This idea has an extremely long and interesting history that originates with the work of Dr. W. Gilman Thompson, who published an article in 1890 on the first efforts to replace neural function by transplantation. Many of these early efforts, not surprisingly, were unsuccessful, but led to a distinguished history of discoveries that now make it possible to attempt neural transplantation in patients.

The Yale work on neurotransplantation began with the discovery in 1985 that the MPTP dopamine-deficit model in primates could be reversed by fetal tissue transplantation.[1] This was followed by methodological issues which now make clinical trials reasonable. First, compared with more developed neural tissue, fetal tissue is unique in its ability to survive transplantation. Second, it retains important capacities after transplantation that might be necessary to restore function. Third, to do a meaningful replacement study, clinical or otherwise, the cells must survive. In order to assure and improve cell survival, we carried out a study of fetal gestational age as a factor associated with survival in the monkey. We found that there is a fetal age that clearly has optimal survival compared with other fetal ages. In the monkey we are confident that we can get significant survival of transplanted cells, which we have illustrated in a number of papers.[3] In a high power photomicrograph, showing the outgrowth of dopamine axons into the surrounding area, one can measure direct increases in dopamine concentrations in the region post mortem. In monkeys that were sham operated or that had cerebellar tissue or older nigral tissue implanted, behavioral recovery occurred only with ideal young nigral tissue. Survival of these extremely impaired monkeys depended upon the appropriate implantation of fetal tissue. They had a much lower probability of survival if they did not have surgery or if they had a sham surgical procedure. The rating of Parkinsonism showed a considerable decrease in the symptoms that were seen based on the appropriate group vs. the inappropriate groups.

Regardless of how persuasive these animal data might be, there are still some very important questions about human patients that are not answered and that cannot be answered with animal studies. The first question is, "will idiopathic Parkinson's disease respond in the same way?" Secondly, "if so and the grafts do survive, how long will they last?" "Will we see graft failure or rejection?" When we first began to confront these issues, we also had to confront questions about the ethics of using fetal tissue and under what circumstances it might be appropriate. We worked out guidelines, which are now widely accepted thanks to the help of many. Still the controversy has not ended and there are, unfortunately, serious protests that continue.

Our next step was to determine if we could successfully implant human fetal tissue in the monkey. After developing the methods to make this possible, and cryopreservation to make it safe and practical,[2] we began our clinical studies in 1988. Our patient groups were similar to those used in Dr. Mahlon DeLong's study. We intended to study classic Parkinson's disease that in uncomplicated by secondary problems. The tissue for transplantation is removed from the area that eventually becomes positive for tyrosine hydroxylase, the enzyme that characterizes neurons that will produce dopamine. Then the tissue is cryopreserved to allow us to schedule the surgery and to accumulate and test tissue before it is implanted into patients. Our group has spent much time developing techniques that will allow implantation to be done effectively and safely. We use magnetic resonance acquired images which are fed into a computer work station that allows the targeting of the areas in the caudate nucleus or the putamen. The tissue is then introduced and implanted. In our first studies, we cautiously implanted only the caudate nucleus on one side; then after the procedure appeared to be safe, the next few patients were implanted on both sides. Most recently, both the caudate and putamen were implanted bilaterally.

We have evaluated patients in a variety of ways. Only one type of rating will be discussed here–videotaped movement examinations which are then analyzed in a blinded and objectively scored fashion, determining both the time required for the task as well as the number of events performed. In these data from our earliest study of unilateral patients, quantitative motor task performance was improved. Patients were capable, for example, of increased number of finger taps within the time period analyzed 18 months after surgery. Continued effects were seen in these three patients from the initial study at three years after surgery. In the standard Parkinson's rating scales, the UPDRS and the Schwab and England scale, there is a consistent pattern of improvement in the patients compared with a control group that did not receive surgery but also had optimized medications. To evaluate the effects of medication, we have also studied our patients in a clinical research unit, off of all anti-parkinson drugs for 48 hours, and repeated every six months after surgery. These data suggest that on the two UPDRS scales (motor and activities of daily living) the patients were improved after surgery off drugs more than they were before while taking their medications. The final effect which has been reported by nearly every group, including ours, is that patients require less anti-parkinson medications to perform at an improved level.[4] All of these studies of medication effects suggest the importance of a strategy to compare transplantation with optimal medication management in order to be sure that the transplant effects are actually better than the best standard treatment. Our "optimized" randomly-assigned control group actually showed some improvements on total UPDRS scores over a one year period, a change that was comparable to some reported transplant effects over the same period.

In conclusion, the importance of determining graft survival if any patients die should be discussed. Without this we will not be able to evaluate and understand any symptom improvement. And we cannot confirm imaging studies that might give us a way to evaluate grafts in living patients in the future. Of our 16 operated patients, all of whom had severe Parkinson's disease, there have been four deaths, and we have obtained autopsy material on three of the four patients.[2] Although we have found evidence for some graft survival, the overall outcome of these autopsies, which we will be reporting in more detail elsewhere, is suggesting that we must continue to watch the immune system, which might be responsible for destroying some grafts and thereby the long-term success of our replacement strategy.

REFERENCES

1. Redmond, D.E., Jr., J.R. Sladek, Jr., R.H. Roth, T.J. Collier, J.D. Elsworth, A.Y. Deutch, and et al., Fetal neuronal grafts in monkeys given methylphenyltetrahydopyridine. Lancet, 1986. i: 125-127.

2. Redmond, D.E., Jr., F. Naftolin, T.J. Collier, C. Leranth, R.J. Robbins, J.D. Sladek et al., Cryopreservation, culture, and transplantation of human fetal mesencephalic tissue into monkeys. Science, 1988. 242:768-771.

3. Redmond, D.E., Jr., R.J. Robbins, F. Naftolin, K.L. Marek, T. Vollmer, C. Leranth et al., Cellular replacement of dopamine deficit in Parkinson's disease using human fetal mesencephalic tissue: Preliminary results in four patients, in Molecular and Cellular Approaches to the Treatment of Brain Disease, S.G. Waxman, Editor. 1993, Raven Press: New York. p. 325-359.

4. Spencer, D.D., R.J. Robbins, F. Naftolin, K.L. Marek, T. Vollmer, C. Leranth, R.H. Roth, L.H. Price, A. Gjedde, B.S. Bunney, K.J. Sass, J.D. Elsworth, E.L. Kier, R. Makuch, P.B. Hoffer, and D.E. Redmond, Jr., Unilateral Transplantation of Human Fetal Mesencephalic Tissue into the Caudate Nucleus of Parkinsonian Patients: Functional Effects for 18 Months. New England Journal of Medicine, 1992. 327:1541-1548.

Proportioned Carbohydrate: Protein Diet in the Management of Parkinson's Disease

M. H. Saint-Hilaire

SUMMARY. The entry of Levodopa into the brain is limited by competition with large neutral amino acids (LNAA). A strict low protein diet improves motor fluctuations but might lead to protein malnutrition. Because insulin secretion lowers plasma LNAA, a stable dietary ratio of carbohydrate:protein might be as effective as protein restriction. This double blind crossover study compared the effects of three proportioned diets: (A) a 7:1 carbohydrate: protein ratio; (B) a 30:1 carbohydrate: protein ratio; and (C) a 1:1.5 carbohydrate:protein ratio, on motor fluctuations, plasma LNAA and levodopa in 12 Parkinson patients. After random assignments to each diet, patients were observed for 11 hours. Serum levodopa and LNAA levels and motor component of the UPDRS were measured hourly. The 7:1 and high carbohydrate diets were both effective at stabilizing plasma LNAA levels. Mean hourly sum of LNAA was significantly different on each of the diets, being highest on the high protein diet and lowest on the high carbohydrate diet. There was a significant correlation between plasma LNAA and amount of "off" time, and a significant inverse correlation between

M. H. Saint-Hilaire, MD, is affiliated with Boston University Medical Center, 80 East Concord Street, C314, Boston, MA 02118.

The author thanks R. G. Feldman, C. A. Thomas, L. M. Perry, and D. L. Turpin who participated in this study and Kristin Boluch for her assistance in manuscript preparation.

Research for this article was supported by a grant from Interneuron Pharmaceuticals, The Harold and Ellen Wald Neurology fund, and the American Parkinson Disease Center of Excellence at Boston University Medical Center.

[Haworth co-indexing entry note]: "Proportioned Carbohydrate: Protein Diet in the Management of Parkinson's Disaese." Saint-Hilaire, M. H. Co-published simultaneously in *Loss, Grief & Care* (The Haworth Press, Inc.) Vol. 8, No. 3/4, 2000, pp. 115-121; and: *Parkinson's Disease and Quality of Life* (ed: Côté et al.) The Haworth Press, Inc., 2000, pp. 115-121. Single or multiple copies of this article are available for a fee from The Haworth Document Delivery Service [1-800-342-9678, 9:00 a.m. - 5:00 p.m. (EST). E-mail address: getinfo@haworthpressinc.com].

115

plasma LNAA and amount of time "on with dyskinesias." A fixed dietary carbohydrate:protein ratio stabilizes plasma LNAA levels and may optimize response to levodopa without the risk of malnutrition. *[Article copies available for a fee from The Haworth Document Delivery Service: 1-800-342-9678. E-mail address: getinfo@haworthpressinc.com]*

Levodopa remains the most effective drug in the treatment of Parkinson's disease (PD) but its long-term use is associated with complications, principally motor fluctuation and abnormal involuntary movements. Motor fluctuations can be partly attributed to the progression of the disease with loss of cells in the substantia nigra and decreased capacity to store dopamine. The clinical response becomes more dependent on plasma levels of levodopa and on efficient passage of levodopa across the blood brain barrier.

The entry of levodopa into the brain is limited by competition with the large neutral amino acids (LNAA) valine, leucine, isoleucine, phenylalanine, tyrosine, and tryptophan, for the transport system.[1] Studies have shown that a diet low in protein improves motor fluctuations.[2,3,4,5] However, the use of low protein diets in PD patients, some of whom are elderly and frail, could lead to protein malnutrition. In addition, it was shown that severe protein restriction below the recommended daily allowance (RDA) is not necessary[6] to affect the clinical response to levodopa. A balanced ratio between carbohydrates and proteins could be as effective in this outcome,[7] because consumption of carbohydrates stimulates insulin secretion, which in turn lowers plasma levels of LNAA.[8] Thus a specific proportion of carbohydrate to protein in the diet may be as effective at stabilizing plasma LNAA levels as reducing the daytime protein intake. The primary objective of this study was to compare the effects of three proportioned carbohydrate to protein diets on motor fluctuations of PD patients. A second objective was to evaluate the effect of each diet on plasma LNAA and levodopa levels.

METHODS

The study was designed as a randomized double blind cross-over trial. Twelve subjects were enrolled after giving informed consent. All were levodopa responders with moderate motor fluctuations (wearing-off or predictable on-off) by history and were Hoehn and Yahr stage 2 or 3 when "on." Patients with weight loss exceeding 5 lbs. in the previous 2 weeks, with diabetes and with unstable renal, hepatic or gastrointestinal disorders were excluded. All patients were taking carbidopa/levodopa (Sinemet) standard and/or controlled release in addition to other antiparkinsonian drugs. The dosage of all medications had been stable for 1 month before entering the study, and remained unchanged during the study, which lasted 4 weeks.

On day one, patients had a physical examination and nutritional assessment, including blood biochemistry. A full United Parkinson Disease Rating Scale (UPDRS)[9] assessment was performed during "on" time. Patients were sent home with instructions to keep a diary of their diet, and to complete two diaries of their motor fluctuations. On those days patients were to record hourly if they were asleep, on without dyskinesias, on with dyskinesias, or "off." During the initial visit patients had been observed and educated about their "on" time, "off" time, and dyskinesias. Two diaries were always completed 6 days and 1 day before each return clinic visit at days 7, 14, 21, and 28. On those days patients were observed for a period of 11 hours in the Parkinson's Day Program at Boston University Medical Center. They arrived in a fasting state prior to their first dose of levodopa. A blood sample was obtained to determine fasting plasma levodopa and LNAA levels. Subjects were given their usual dose of levodopa at 7:15 a.m. and continued on their regular antiparkinsonian medications schedule for the rest of the day. Serum levels of LNAA and levodopa were measured, and clinical evaluations were performed hourly until 5:15 p.m. Clinical evaluation consisted of the motor component of the UPDRS, and recording of dyskinesias and "on" and "off" states. The full UPDRS was done once during each clinic visit when patients were "on." On day 7 patients received a standardized breakfast and lunch containing a 7:1 carbohydrate: protein ration at 8:15 a.m. and 1:15 p.m. At the end of that day patients were sent home with one of three randomized test drinks. The first drink (7:1) contained a fixed 7:1 carbohydrate: protein ratio; the second drink (HC) contained a 30:1 carbohydrate: protein ratio; and the third drink (HP) contained a 1.5:1 carbohydrate: protein ratio. The caloric content of each beverage was 470Kcal/package. The 7:1 drink contained 12.2g protein/package; the HC drink contained 3.1g protein/package; and the HP drink contained 38.1g protein/package. The content of the package was diluted in 12 oz. of water before consumption. Patients were instructed to take one package for breakfast and lunch and suggestions were made for snacks and balanced evening meals. Snacks respected the proportion of carbohydrate:protein the patients were receiving in the test drink. When patients returned to the clinic on days 14, 21 and 28, the test beverage was given for breakfast and lunch. At the end of days 14 and 21 another test drink was randomly distributed so that by the end of the study, all patients had received each of the test drinks for 1 week.

Serum levodopa was measured by HPLC with electrochemical detection.[10] Plasma tryptophan was measured using the fluorometric method of Denkla and Dewey.[11] LNAA was analyzed by ion exchange chromatography with Ninhydrin detection using the Beckman Spherogel Amino Acid column and corresponding lithium and Ninhydrin reagents. The HPLC equipment included a spectra physics system to which had been added a Beckman

System gold Ninhydrin pump, column heater and post column reactor.[12] The data was entered and verified in SAS data sets, ANOVA was used to analyze change from baseline for variables described. Duncan's Multiple Range Tests were conducted on treatment means to determine where significant differences existed when the ANOVA showed significant treatment effects.

RESULTS

Data analyses were conducted on the results obtained from 10 evaluable patients. One patient was noncompliant with beverage consumption and one patient withdrew after his second treatment regimen because he felt that his functional status was declining.

Clinical performance. Average time "on" or "on with dyskinesias" was 78% on the 7:1 drink, 81% on the HC drink, and 68% on the HP drink. The average time "on with dyskinesias" 42% on the 7:1 drink, 48% on the HC drink and 25% on the HP drink. None of the numbers are statistically different, but the data suggest there is more "off" time with the high protein diet and more time "on with dyskinesias" on the high carbohydrate diet. There was no significant difference in the total UPDRS score, nor in each part of the UPDRS, when "on," on each of the diets. The patient diary data did not show statistically significant differences among treatments for percentage "on" time of awake hours.

The area under the curve for the motor score of the UPDRS was significantly greater (215.60 ± 105.76) on the HP drink than on the other drinks. There was no significant difference between the AUC on the 7:1 drink (167.35 ± 96.34) and the HC drink (182.05 ± 99.03).

Plasma LNAA and levodopa levels. The mean hourly sum of LNAA was 576 ± 60nM/ml on the 7:1 drink, 441 ± 51nM/ml on the HC drink and 966 ± 212nM/ml on the HP drink. The LNAA levels were all statistically significantly different from each other (p < 0.05, on way ANOVA using Newman Keuls multiple mean comparison). There was a significant difference in the AUC for LNAA on each of the diets. AUC was 4594.6 ± 346 on the 7:1 drink, 3501 ± 612.3 on the HC drink and 7878.6 ± 615.4 on the HP drink.

Baseline LNAA level was not significantly different at 7:00 a.m. on each day of the study, but subsequent levels were significantly higher on the HP drink. Serum LNAA levels were significantly lower after breakfast and lunch on the HC drink compared to the 7:1 drink. This seems to indicate that LNAA levels are less variable on the 7:1 drink, decreased on the HC drink and increased on the HP drink.

Mean hourly Levodopa level was 1.0 ± 0.45 mcg/ml on the 7:1 drink, 0.89 ± 0.41 mcg/ml on the HC drink and 0.96 ± 0.33 mcg/ml on HP drink. These levels were not significantly different. The AUC for levodopa was also not significantly different on each of the diets. AUC was 7.9 ± 3.8 on the 7:1 drink, 7.2 ± 3.5 on the HC drink and 7.5 ± 3 on the HP drink.

Levodopa flux. A relative levodopa flux was calculated using the equation.[1]

Levodopa flux was significantly lower on the HP drink (0.0854 ± 0.0342) than on the two other drinks. There was no significant difference between the flux on the 7:1 drink (0.1511 ± 0.0712) and the flux on the HC drink (0.1857 ± 0.0888).

Correlation between clinical response and serum LNAA levels. Although there was no significant difference in the amount of time "on" and "off" on each of the diets, there was a significant ($p < 0.018$, $r^2 = 0.999$) correlation between mean LNAA levels and percent time "off." As the mean LNAA level increased, the time "off" increased. No significant correlation was found with mean LNAA level and percent of time spent just "on," but there was a significant inverse correlation ($p < 0.003$, $r^2 = 0.999$) between mean LNAA and percent of time spent "on with dyskinesias."

DISCUSSION

It is now well established that levodopa competes with plasma LNAA for absorption across the blood brain barrier.[1] This has been shown by Positron Emission Tomography[13] and by demonstrating that administration of LNAA to Parkinsonian patients stabilized on a constant infusion of levodopa worsened motor signs.[4] A low protein or protein redistribution diet can improve clinical response to levodopa with increase "on" time in patients with "on-off" phenomenon.[2,3,5,14,16,17] The benefit from the diet appears to persist after long-term follow-up in most patients.[18] However, most studies have been short-term and have focused on a total protein restriction to 0.5/kg/day[14] or on a daytime restriction to less than 7g before the evening meal.[5,16] An eight week study[19] of Parkinsonian patients on a daytime restricted protein diet showed a significant decrease in their protein, calcium and iron intake, although this resulted in little change in their body weight. Subjects had difficulties increasing their intake of protein at the evening meal to compensate for the restriction during the day, suggesting that protein restriction can compromise nutrition in certain patients with inadequate diets. In addition, it has been found that 52% of patients with Parkinson's disease have significant weight loss anyway, despite protein and caloric intake in the recommended range.[20]

Our data show that a stringent daytime protein restriction is not necessary to stabilize blood levels of LNAA if there is a balanced ratio of carbohydrates to protein. A higher carbohydrate intake raises plasma insulin, reduces plasma LNAA and elevates the ratio of dopa to LNAA. Intake of protein on the

7:1 carbohydrate: protein diet was 24.5g during the daytime, which is still restricted but significantly higher than the 7g or less recommended on the strict redistribution diet. However, LNAA levels were more stable on this ratio than on the more restricted diet which was associated with a trend to lower LNAA levels, and potential increased incidence of dyskinesias as the day goes on.

Serum levels of levodopa did not differ on each of the diets, demonstrating again that protein intake does not interfere with the gastrointestinal absorption of levodopa[3,5] and the competition for active transport in the intestine is probably negligible. Lowering serum LNAA levels is more crucial in promoting delivery of levodopa to the brain, improving levodopa flux as shown in our study and Carter's study.[3]

There was no significant increase in duration of "on" time on the high carbohydrate diet and the 7:1 ratio diet compared to the high protein diet. This is probably due to the small number of patients, and the fact that our patients were predictable fluctuators and would not benefit as much from a low protein diet as severe fluctuators with unpredictable on-off.[18] However, we could demonstrate the strong relationship between serum LNAA levels and the clinical response to levodopa. Low levels of LNAA are associated with more dyskinesias, and as the levels increase, "off" time is also increased. This supports the importance of maintaining serum LNAA levels as stable as possible especially in patients with severe fluctuations and dyskinesias. Our study shows that a 7:1 carbohydrate:protein ratio in the diet can stabilize LNAA levels, and a previous study[7] reported similar results with a 5:1 ratio. Further studies will have to address which ratio is optimal to maintain predictable plasma LNAA levels. The long-term nutritional impact of such a diet must also be studied, as the ultimate goal of nutritional intervention in PD is to prevent protein, vitamin, mineral and caloric malnutrition in addition to minimizing primary and secondary symptoms of the disease.

REFERENCES

1. Pardridge W. Regulation of amino acid availability to the brain. In: Wurtman RJ, Wurtman JJ, eds. Nutrition and the brain: New York: Raven Press, 1977:141-204.

2. Pincus JH, Barr K. Influence of dietary protein on motor fluctuations in Parkinson's Disease. Arch Neurol 1987;44:270-272.

3. Carter JH, Nutt JG, Woodward WR, Hatcher LF, Trotman TL. Amount and distribution of dietary protein affects clinical response to levodopa in Parkinson's Disease. Neurology 1989;39:552-556.

4. Nutt JH, Woodward W, Hammerstad JP, Carter JH, Anderson JL. The on-off phenomenon in Parkinson's disease. Relation to levodopa absorption and transport. N Engl J Med 1984; 310:483-488.

5. Tsui JK, Ross S, Poulin K, Douglas J, Postnikoff D, Calne S, Woodward W, Calne DB. The effect of dietary protein on the efficacy of L-Dopa. A double blind study. Neurology 1989;39:549-552.

6. Juncos DL, Fabbrini G, Mouradian MM, Serrati C, Chase TN. Dietary influences on the antiparkinsonian response to levodopa. Arch Neurol 1987;44:1003-1005.

7. Berry EM, Growdon JH, Wurtman JJ, Caballero B, Wurtman RJ. A balanced carbohydrate: protein diet in the management of Parkinson's disease. Neurology 1991;41:1295-1297.

8. Wurtman R, Caballero B, Salzman E. Facilitation of levodopa-induced dyskinesias by dietary carbohydrates. N Engl J Med 1988;319:1288-1289.

9. Fahn S, Elton RL. Unified Parkinson's Disease rating scale. In: Fahn S, Marsden CD, Calne DB, Goldstein M, eds. Recent development in Parkinson's disease, Vol III. Florham Park, NJ: MacMillan, 1987:153-163.

10. Titus DC, August TF. Simultaneous HPLC analysis of carbidopa, levodopa and 3-0 methyldopa in plasma. J of Chromatography 1990;534:87-100.

11. Denkla WD, Dewey HK. The determination of tryptophan in plasma, liver, and urine. J Lab Clin Med 1967;69:160-169.

12. Armstrong, MD, and Stave, U. A study of plasma free amino acid levels. II. Normal values for children and adults. Metabolism 1973;22:561-569.

13. Leenders KL, Poewe WH, Palmer AJ, Brenton DP, Fraackowiak RSJ. Inhibition of L-[18F] Fluorodopa uptake into human brain by amino-acids demonstrated by positron emission tomography. Ann Neurol 1986, 20:258-262.

14. Riley D, Lang AE. Practical application of a low-protein diet for Parkinson's disease. Neurology 1988;38:1026-1031.

15. Mena I, Cotzias G. Protein intake and treatment of Parkinson's disease with levodopa. N Engl J Med 1975;292:181-184.

16. Pincus JH, Barry KM. Plasma levels of Amino acids correlate with motor fluctuations in Parkinsonism. Arch Neurol 1987;44:1006-1009.

17. Eriksson T, Granérus AK, Linde A, Carlsson A. On-off phenomenon in Parkinson's disease: relationship between dopa and other large neutral amino acids in plasma. Neurology 1988;38:1245-1248.

18. Karstaldt P, Pincus JH. Protein redistribution diet remains effective in patients with fluctuating parkinsonism. Arch Neurol 1992;49:149-151.

19. Paré S, Barr SI, Ross SE. Effect of daytime protein restriction on nutrient intakes of free-living Parkinson's Disease patients. Am J Clin Nutr 1992;55:701-707.

20. Abbott RA, Cox M, Markus H, Tomkins A. Diet, body size and micronutrient status in Parkinson's disease. Eur J of Clin Nutr 1992;46:879-884.

On Being an Advocate
for Parkinson's Disease Research

Joan Samuelson

There are many times when it is very obvious that I have Parkinson's disease. I was diagnosed eight years ago. In 1990 I read in the paper about the possible promise of a breakthrough for Parkinson's, a substantial breakthrough in tissue transplant therapy. I was caught with a surge of excitement and hope that I hadn't felt in a long time which was then swept away by the frustration of reading on about the federal policy banning any federal support for that research in the United States because of the connection to its use of tissue from elective abortions. From those emotions, I eventually formed this organization because it became clear that we needed a voice in Washington that would speak on our behalf to talk about the terrible price of Parkinson's and the desperate need for every obstacle in our way to be lifted so that we could get a cure as soon as possible. I went, with others, to Washington, spoke about our story, testified in hearings, met with congressmen and senators, and after a brutal fight of 2 1/2 years we finally got the ban lifted. It was a terrible fight in the Congress. We won an overwhelming majority of both houses of Congress but President Bush vetoed the bill. Our effort to override the veto was overwhelmingly supported in the senate, but we lost by eleven votes in the house. Then President Clinton lifted the ban on his second day in office. At the signing ceremony, President Clinton told our Chair, Ann Udal, that while he was on the campaign trail, he was profoundly moved when he heard from people around the country who had Parkinson's and who came up to him and said such things as "please help us by lifting the ban," and "by the way, Governor Clinton, I would never vote for you, except for this, and I'm going to vote for you because of it."

Joan Samuelson, Esquire, is affiliated with Parkinson's Action Network, Santa Rosa, CA.

[Haworth co-indexing entry note]: "On Being an Advocate for Parkinson's Disease Research." Samuelson, Joan. Co-published simultaneously in *Loss, Grief & Care* (The Haworth Press, Inc.) Vol. 8, No. 3/4, 2000, pp. 123-125; and: *Parkinson's Disease and Quality of Life* (ed: Côté et al.) The Haworth Press, Inc., 2000, pp. 123-125. Single or multiple copies of this article are available for a fee from The Haworth Document Delivery Service [1-800-342-9678, 9:00 a.m. - 5:00 p.m. (EST). E-mail address: getinfo@haworthpressinc.com].

123

From that moment on, our mission changed quite a bit. While we were working in Washington those first couple of years, we became quite impressed and, at the same time, horrified with the fact of how the system worked. Earlier panelists have talked about the difficulty of going to people, our friends and loved ones as well as well as colleagues and acquaintances, and saying "Hi, I have Parkinson's." I had that same difficulty, so I fully understand the difficulty of it. But what I saw in Washington, overwhelmingly so, was people swarming Capital Hill and the rest of DC saying "Hi, I'm (so and so) and I have (blank)." I have cancer. I have Alzheimer's. I have multiple sclerosis. I have AIDS. I have breast cancer. And there seemed to be this direct correlation. They would say what disease they had and they would receive money. There is a chart that compares the amount of money spent per patient for various diseases. Of course, some diseases have a much bigger population than we do. We showed the total money spent, the number of patients, and a cost-per-patient comparison. Parkinson's disease is simply at the bottom of the list. The federal government spends $30.00 per patient per year. Thirty dollars for each person with Parkinson's on research to cure this disease. That is awful. The other awful thing is to see that they spend a lot more for other diseases. Those people need it, too. They are suffering and/or dying, too, and the money is well spent, but we should be getting the same amount of money as well. Since the lifting of the ban, we have been talking about the wider picture of Parkinson's research and the enormous potential in many areas. One part of this work that had been very exciting for me personally is talking to scientists around the country, many of whom have a passion for a particular area: fetal transplants; pallidotomies; genetic testing; genetic therapies; gene therapies; neural growth factor (where they think they may be able to send in something that will change the gene or somehow give a message to get those dopamine cells running again). I would be very excited and then the scientist would say "Boy, but I could be much more aggressive about this research if I had a bigger staff, if I had a better lab, if I simply could get a federal grant at all so that I could do more than one teeny clinical trial." That became our job.

What we are doing now is a combination of things to make that happen. The most wonderful thing about the last year was the decision by Senator Hatfield and Congressman Waxman, who have become dedicated champions for Parkinson's research, to introduce a bill specifically on our behalf, the Morris K. Udall Parkinson's Research and Education Act. It is named after Mo Udall, who was in congress for thirty years and was forced to retire in 1991 due to advanced Parkinson's disease. Mo Udall was much loved and is missed in Congress and people immediately make the connection from his name to Parkinson's disease and the need to break through and cure it. Members of his family, especially his daughter Ann, have been enormously helpful in working with the Congressmen to spread awareness. While the bill is pending, we are also working on initiating the appropriations process. The budget and federal funding are very tight. It has been a terribly hard struggle but the bottom line is that other disorders have been able to work hard and get the money they need. The success story that I look to as a model is the Alzheimer's community.

Ten years ago, the Alzheimer's community had ten million dollars a year in federal research funding for Alzheimer's. The Alzheimer's advocates became active. They went to Capitol Hill. They started talking about their cause. They started talking about their loved ones. They started telling their personal story, which is an extremely effective technique. There is an image of Washington as being full of very, very slick men, and sometimes women, in businesses and briefcases, approaching congressmen to talk about their companies and their need for dollars to go to certain industries. However, I have also seen the impact of ordinary people telling their stories and making those members cry. And we've done it. It isn't just the afflicted person. After the first hearing in the Senate on the fetal tissue campaign, the staffs of the members of the committee talked about how powerful it was to have one witness after another telling their stories. There were staff people walking out of the room because they couldn't stop crying and there were tears in the eyes of some of the senators. One of the staff members said "You know, that's right, you all had us just absolutely in tears . . . but the other thing that was so overwhelming was to see your husband there in that row right behind you with tears in his eyes as well." My husband will turn around in a room when he starts talking about the impact on our marriage and his fears of the future. It is very powerful and it works.

It has been helpful to me to feel that there was something I could do for myself and for my husband and for other members of my family who have gone out and buttonholed their own congressman. We desperately need your help. Any helpful bill is just a piece of paper. That is all it is until a majority of the two houses of Congress pass it, the President signs it, it receives appropriations and the NIH actually does it. That is where everyone can be an advocate. Each of us has the power to use. Professional support staff to the Parkinson's community have seen stories and know people who are afflicted with Parkinson's. People afflicted by Parkinson's can tell their stories. Caregivers of loved ones or acquaintances or professional colleagues of someone with PD can talk about how it has ripped a person's life apart or how terribly it has impacted their careers. Everyone has a story. One of the wonderful things we try to do is to bring scientists and physicians in who can talk about the promise of their work and their frustration with not having enough money to find a cure so that the suffering can end, and the cost of caring for people with Parkinson's can end, because they will be able to return to work, pay taxes and so on. I implore everyone to get involved.

How to Get Organized as a Caregiver

Gloria A. Scherma

WANTED:
PEOPLE WILLING TO ACCEPT THE JOB OF A CAREGIVER

What is a caregiver? One who, without monetary compensation, physically cares for an impaired relative; spouse, parent, child, other relative or significant other. A caregiver usually has been emotionally involved with the impaired person prior to the impaired persons disability, and is most frequently an older woman.

HELP WANTED AD

Wanted: a person willing to work all hours of the day, seven days a week, no vacation, personal days or holidays. There is no salary, bonuses, 401K plans. There is no supervisor or on the job training and no yearly Christmas party. You must be emotionally involved with the person you are going to work for and be willing to work until you are physically exhausted. You must be self starter and an entrepreneur. You must also be willing to learn the job by trial and error. The person you are going to care for will probably become more impaired and frequently will not be able to express any appreciation and may even be abusive to you. Anyone interested in this job, apply immediately.

No one in their right mind would want this job! However, whole armies of people have accepted this responsibility. Frequently, people have no choice.

Gloria A. Scherma, MPS, is affiliated with Multi-Comprehensive Consulting Services, Inc., 1618 West 3rd Street, Brooklyn, NY 11223.

[Haworth co-indexing entry note]: "How to Get Organized as a Caregiver." Scherma, Gloria A. Co-published simultaneously in *Loss, Grief & Care* (The Haworth Press, Inc.) Vol. 8, No. 3/4, 2000, pp. 127-134; and: *Parkinson's Disease and Quality of Life* (ed: Côté et al.) The Haworth Press, Inc., 2000, pp. 127-134. Single or multiple copies of this article are available for a fee from The Haworth Document Delivery Service [1-800-342-9678, 9:00 a.m. - 5:00 p.m. (EST). E-mail address: getinfo@haworthpressinc.com].

More commonly, people accept this responsibility because they honestly care for the person for whom they are caring. How then, does one tackle this job, become a proficient competent caregiver, without experiencing total burnout and maintaining one's sanity on the job? One of the most efficient ways to function as a caregiver is to organize and keep information on all the issues affecting the impaired person. This article takes the caregiver through the first steps of organizing that information.

The first thing you will have to do is to purchase the following:

- A large loose leaf book
- Several packages of loose leaf paper
- Section dividers with pockets
- Two calendars (one for appointments and one for Reality Orientation—see section on Reality Orientation)
- Colored pens
- Labels

The sections in the loose leaf book should be as follows:

1. Personal Information
2. Family and Friends
3. Insurance
4. Health Information/Medical Professionals
5. Home Safety Analysis
6. Researching Home Health Agencies/Hiring an Aide
7. Legal Issues
8. Financial Issues
9. Final Arrangements
10. Home Service and Repair Numbers
11. Reality Orientation
12. Local Resources
13. Take Care of Yourself
14. Using the Workbook

On the outside of the loose leaf book affix a label that states this book belongs to (and state the name of the person) and should be used in case of an emergency.

The following is information that should be included in each section:

1. Personal Information

A. Identification: Name, address, telephone number, date of birth, religion, religious leader, house of worship, location

B. Emergency information: Police number 911 and the local precinct number, fire department local number, Poison Control Center number, ipecac location

C. Known allergies

2. Family and Friends

A. Name, address, work and home phone number for the primary person responsible for the impaired person.

B. Emergency back-up numbers; who is next in line to call in case of an emergency.

C. Name, address, phone number of nearest neighbor.

D. Name, address, phone number of all other relatives or friends that could be involved with this person.

3. Insurance Information

A. Medical Insurance: Medicare number (make a copy of the Medicare card and keep it in the book), Medicare supplemental number, other insurance

B. Life Insurance policy number, amount, company, beneficiary, name and number of agent who wrote the policy, if possible

C. Disability policy

D. Household insurance: Record the location of all of the above documents

4. Health Information/Medical Professionals

A. Existing medical condition: Medications (in original containers and clearly marked). Schedule for medications. Name, address, telephone number of local pharmacist that delivers. Name, address, phone number of the primary physician, and the medications that are prescribed. Name, address, phone numbers for all other specialists, and the medications they prescribe.

B. Name, address, phone numbers for physical therapist and occupational therapist (if appropriate).

C. Name, address, phone number for their dentist and if necessary one who makes house calls.

D. Name, address, phone number of their ophthalmologist as well as the name, address, phone number of the optometrist.

E. Name, address, telephone number for durable medical equipment (hospital bed, walkers, commodes, etc.).

F. Name, address, telephone number of local handyman to make necessary modifications in the home (grab bars in the bathroom, ramp for wheelchair, etc.).

G. Conduct a food analysis, what does the patient like to eat and when?

H. If the patient was recently discharged from the hospital, include a copy of the patient's discharge plan.

I. If the patient is to be visited by Visiting Nurse Services, the address, phone number, and name of the team coordinator.

J. Have sign-in sheets for all professional, progress notes, and medication schedules in the book as well.

K. Have the following document signed: Authorization for emergency care; emergency information; medication authorization; health care proxy.

5. Home Safety Analysis

A. The primary person responsible for the care of the impaired person should check the home for possible hazards and eliminate all hazardous elements.

B. Start with the entrance: does the door have secure locks and does the home need an alarm that connects to the police department?

C. Check all the flooring: Are there rugs that need to be made skid proof or removed? Are there door saddles that make walking difficulty? Are the floors so highly polished that they are slippery?

D. Check the kitchen: Are the chairs sturdy enough to support the patient? Does the patient need a chair with arms? Is the table a good height to eat from? Does the patient need special eating implements, or reaching implements? Is the stove gas and does it light properly? Would it be best to purchase a microwave and eliminate the danger of a regular stove? Is the stove free from any debris (saved plastic bags, paper plates, etc.)?

E. Check all windows: Are they secure? Do they need screens? Do they need bars for safety?

F. Check the bathroom: Does the tub have a non-skid surface, decals or rug to prevent falls? Does the patient need a bathing stool and hand held shower? Does the patient need grab bars around the tub and around the toilet? Does the patient need a high-hat toilet seat to make using the toilet easier? Does the patient need new and larger bath towels to properly be wrapped in after bathing to prevent chills?

G. Check the bedroom: Is the bed comfortable or does the patient need a hospital bed, an egg crate or an adjustable bed? Does the patient need side-rails for the existing bed? Does the patient have appropriate linens? Is there a non-skid rug next to the bed?

H. Check the living room? Are the chairs comfortable for the patient to sit in? Where does the patient like to read, watch television? Is there adequate lighting?

I. Check the stairways: Are they adequately lighted? Are they free from clutter and loose objects? Is there a secure bannister or sturdy hand-rail?

J. Are all electric cords placed close to the wall and in good condition?

K. Are flashlights strategically placed about the home?

L. Does the patient need a safety alarm system, and if so, what type would be best suited for the patient?

6. Researching Home Health Agencies/Hiring an Aide

A. Call several agencies to obtain necessary information for comparisons. Rates vary greatly. Choose a home care agency with great care, this is may be one of the most important decisions you can make. Don't hesitate to ask questions and lots of them.

B. If your friends or other family members have used a home health care agency, ask them to tell you the pros and cons of their experiences.

C. Check with your local hospital's Social Service Department for the names of recommended home health care agencies.

D. When you have narrowed your selection, check with the local Better Business Bureau to see if there have been any consumer complaints registered against the agency.

E. It's a good idea to have the patient involved in the interviewing process before you make a final decision regarding an aide.

Questions to Ask the Home Health Agency

- How long has the agency been in existence?
- How are the home health aides recruited?
- What is the length of their training and experience?
- Does the agency have references for each aide?
- When are the aides available? Days? Nights? Weekends?
- Is care available on a live-in basis? Part-time? Full-time?
- How far in advance do arrangements have to be made?
- Do aides have their own cars or do they rely on public transportation after a certain night-time hour? Will you have to pay for their car-fare?
- Are aides paid directly by you or through the agency?
- What are the aides' duties?
- If you are dissatisfied with the assigned aide, will a substitute be available?
- Do live-ins have to have their own rooms?

- During what hours is the agency available to receive calls?
- Is an administrator from the agency available 24 hours a day, seven days a week?
- What is the aide's record of punctuality and attendance?
- What are the minimum and maximum hours that can be arranged?
- Are the aides licensed and/or bonded?

7. Legal Issues

A. Record the name, address, telephone number of the patient's attorney.
B. If there is a will make sure you have a copy, and the attorney has a copy.
C. Is the will current or does it need to be updated?
D. Record the name, address, and telephone number of the executor of the estate.
E. Are there minor children that will require a guardian?
F. Should the patient establish a Contingency Trust for Minors?
G. Does the patient want to establish a Marital or Non-Marital Trust?
H. Have you moved and is the will relevant in the state you are currently living in?
I. Obtain a Durable Power of Attorney.
J. Is there is a sizable estate? You might want to talk to an attorney who specializes in elder law issues.

8. Financial Issues

A. Record the names, addresses, telephone numbers. contact people for banking institutes.
B. Record the names, addresses, telephone numbers of any investment advisors.
C. Record savings accounts; checking accounts, CD's; other investments.
D. Record all pensions, social security checks, etc. Arrange for direct deposit.
E. Safe deposit location, number, location of keys.
F. Some institutes require their own documentation for Durable Powers of Attorney.
G. Have joint accounts with your name or another responsible person's name on the account as well as the patient's name.

9. Final Arrangements

A. Steps to take when someone dies.
- Report death (usually the hospital or attending doctor attends to this detail).

- Request several copies of the Death Certificate (you will need it to notify all institutes; banks, investments, social security, real estate, etc.).
- Check with the deceased's former employer or union (pensions, continued health benefits for the spouse, an annuity, etc.).
- Call all credit card companies.
- If there is a home loan or mortgage, notify the bank and remove the name of the deceased. Do the same if you have homeowner's insurance.
- Notify creditors. If you are the administrator of the estate, you are responsible for settling all debts.
- Verify all questionable bills that come in after the death of a person.

10. Home Service and Repair Numbers

A. Record all service and repair numbers; telephone, utilities, exterminator, electrician, dry cleaners, laundry, food delivery, newspaper, handyman, plumber, roofer, security system, carpenter, cable television, etc.
B. Record the locations of household items; electrical fuse box, gas meter, main water valves, thermostats, septic tank, furnace, telephone control box, etc.
C. Record where home supplies are kept; extra paper products, medicines/first aid, lighting supplies, cleaning/laundry supplies, etc.

11. Reality Orientation

A. Put a calendar within easy view of the patient, and use the calendar for the following:
  - Mark all important dates for all family and friends (use different colored pens for different occasions) birthdays, anniversaries, national holidays. It is important to keep the patient in touch with as many things as you can. Discuss the weather, what kinds of clothing you have to wear, the seasons, time of day, etc.

12. Local Resources

A. Record the names, addresses, telephone numbers of agencies that at some time may be able to assist you: Department for the Aging, Meals on Wheels, Social Security, Respite Services, Frail Centers, Social Services, Friendly Visitors Services, etc.

13. Take Care of Yourself

Remember that you are the most important person in this household. You must remember to take care of yourself. Ask friends, relatives, religious associates, neighbors, to relieve you on a regular basis, not just when you are so exhausted that you are ready to collapse. Try to arrange for respite services, so that you can have some extended time for yourself. Take time to go for a walk, take a hot bath, read a book, go to dinner with a friend, take a drive, buy yourself a gift; some flowers, a book, etc. You must, must, must take care of yourself!!

14. Using the Workbook

Initially you will use the workbook to enter all the data mentioned above. After you have entered the data, use the workbook to keep all relevant information about the patient. If you get in the habit of using one book instead of writing things on scraps of paper and then having to look for them, you will always have all the information you need right at your fingertips. Use the pockets of the dividers to keep loose papers, receipts, etc. As both a gerontologist with a private practice and a caregiver, I live with these issues everyday, both as a professional and as a caregiver. I wish all my fellow caregivers the best of luck, and will hold all of you in my prayers.

Effects of Parkinson's Disease (PD) on Family Life

Lola L. Sprinzeles

Chronic disease is a condition which produces an infinite variety of effects upon family interaction accentuated by the personality of each person within the family, the emotional approach towards one another and the family as a unit. PD is a progressive neurological movement disorder with permanent chronicity. Although the etiology is not known, research abounds and Fahn et al. (1992) strongly believe that free radicals influence the development of PD. Various factors affect the perception of disease and the adaptation of coping mechanism, declared Wright (1959). For example, individual differences and premorbid personality of patient and family members, the functional role within the familial hierarchy, physical, mental and social aspects, age of onset, the type of neurological condition and stage of disease process, pathology, disabling sequelae, trauma, heredity, probability of recovery or improvement, economic solvency, solidity of the family constellation, availability of support systems, and ability to use them, cultural attitudes, etc., to name a few. Some criteria may not specifically apply to PD or to particular patients and their families, but some general principles pertain to the effect on family life of all (neurological) disabilities.

PD is not known to occur at birth, is very rare in childhood, but according to Langston (1992) may develop in early adulthood, and strikes most often in midlife or later. Each age group presents its own characteristics and problems, requiring different adaptations. There are also cultural differences. In the Occident and Mideast, personal values are rooted in body image and

Lola L. Sprinzeles, PhD, CRC, RN, is Clinical Specialist, Research, Advocacy, and Counseling, Parkinson's Disease Foundation, Columbia-Presbyterian Center, New York Presbyterian Hospital, New York, NY.

[Haworth co-indexing entry note]: "Effects of Parkinson's Disease (PD) on Family Life." Sprinzeles, Lola L. Co-published simultaneously in *Loss, Grief & Care* (The Haworth Press, Inc.) Vol. 8, No. 3/4, 2000, pp. 135-142; and: *Parkinson's Disease and Quality of Life* (ed: Côté et al.) The Haworth Press, Inc., 2000, pp. 135-142. Single or multiple copies of this article are available for a fee from The Haworth Document Delivery Service [1-800-342-9678, 9:00 a.m. - 5:00 p.m. (EST). E-mail address: getinfo@haworthpressinc.com].

perfection. Conversely, impairment produces a negative self-concept and non-visible disability is denied. Wright (1959) asserted that youth oriented and "body-beautiful" conscious societies do not easily tolerate handicaps. Therefore, when disability strikes an individual, it tends to produce stress. The now disabled person and/or the family are tempted to hide the impediment. However, public education may dispel negative consequences such as rejection or personal and social discrimination or premature termination of employment due to social non-acceptance. As Strong (1988) indicated physical and psychic energies used for denial could be more advantageously applied to the acquisition of positive adaptive coping mechanisms. Anticipation of adversities may cause undue anxiety in the parties involved. Compounding the issue is imposed or self-selected social isolation. While patients may seek gratification of dependency needs and increase the family's plight, Flapan (1989) warns caregivers against total immersion in patientcare to the exclusion of other interests. Then too, people may feel embarrassed of not conforming with "social" norms; harbor guilt and resentment about negative consequences of disability; have fear and guilt of possible heredity passed on to one's descendents; or, in case of family history of neurological disorders, rage towards one's own parent(s). Genetic counseling may help people understand and cope with these feelings. Children and/or spouses may resent having to relinquish normal leisure-time pleasures; or having been cheated of one's anticipated "trouble free" retirement; or be angry for having to change professional pursuits (usually because of additional financial or temporal demands, as Mace et al. (1981) proclaimed); some people feel ashamed of their disabled family member; resent additional tasks in an already crowded schedule or have other limitations imposed on them.

Once a permanent disabling condition is manifested, the family may have to demonstrate an inordinate amount of selflessness to maintain a semblance of family life. Usually, such situations are most difficult for the spouse because of inherent expectations of sacrifice of one's life over and beyond the demands on others within the society. Not all people enter a relationship with such a high degree of dedication; but in many ways the non-impaired partner in marriage may face more serious issues than the spouse. While in most families emotional stability must exist to confront the future with equanimity, in some situations, such selflessness may be questioned for evidence of psychological pathology of the non-disabled person. Often, professional intervention such as individual and/or group psychotherapy, social work or pastoral counseling and/or support groups help people cope better. Yalom (1981) expounds the therapeutic benefit of groups. It is noteworthy that a higher percentage of counseling arises in families of disabled men. The most frequently reported reasons for friction are: (1) economic pressure because in most cases, the man is the primary breadwinner; and (2) sexual dysfunction affirmed by Lipe et al. (1990). (Western) society is more readily prepared to tolerate non-employment and/or sexual passivity in women than in men. Moreover, it is more acceptable for women to cry and release pent-up emotions. Tears tend to "wash away" pain and stimulate the production of endorphins which are biogenic amines with analgesic properties. Women's disability tends to be less disruptive to the family and is discussed in later pages.

Strauss, P. (1994) argues that the poor are covered medically for various eventualities, and the affluent have the means to pay their expenses, but the middle class is often economically depleted from the effects of chronic disease. (Some spouses divorce their marital partners primarily because of finances. Once divorced, legally financial liability for the disabled mate has ceased.)

Patients and families must be helped to acquire (more) effective coping mechanisms. Strauss, A. (1984) recommends counseling with or without the disabled individual to clarify misconceptions about a disorder and to afford an opportunity to re-examine the adjustments that have been made, or need to be made, within the family, if the family is to continue as a unit. Counseling provides also a stage wherein family members can examine their reaction to a particular situation which has to be faced. Family members, only too often, perceive their emotions as socially unacceptable. They are convinced that society condemns them for not willingly foregoing maintenance or establishment of meaningful relationships with others or wanting to participate in social activities available to those who do not have to "care for" disabled family members. The non-disabled individuals may attempt to avoid acknowledging these feelings which are of themselves natural and part of the human condition and, by repressing them, produce an anxiety that they themselves do not understand. Garrett (1952) poses several questions. What does one do when a disabled person is perceived to enjoy the dependency and lack of responsibility? Are the non-disabled to deny their own perceptions? Are they aware there are secondary gains from a disability? On the other hand, the non-disabled may consciously or subliminally derive satisfaction from control over the disabled or feel grateful not being the neuropathic victim; and the impaired person may be angry with the "healthy" one for his/her personal well-being, and covertly, if not overtly, become more burdensome as a means of expressing resentment.

Therapy and/or support groups are often effective means of coping with disability. Drawn from her own experience as psychotherapist and support group leader, Sprinzeles (1994) dealt with groups of varied compositions. Groups may be permanently or intermittently homogeneous; one may consist of patients; one of family members; or the groups may be combined. Still others may alternate their group format. Counseling the impaired individual together with members of the family can teach all concerned how to communicate honestly and share their feelings of perhaps being manipulated by others, of having needs and desires that are diametrically opposed, etc. Stress, anxiety and tension are present in everybody's life and are normal occurrences; but they are frequently more difficult to acknowledge when one family member is impaired. Methods of dealing with them determine the degree of adjustment or maladjustment one reaches.

In Western society the nuclear family is normally responsible for the care of the disabled member, often with assistance from the community. In Middle Eastern cultures, the vastly extended family or "clan" is expected to supplement the ministrations of the immediate family. Should a member of the family become disabled, the burden of caring is shared by many. In contrast, Oriental cultures view disability as a natural phenomenon with less tendency to hide the impairment. A reference by Buck (1950) to a disabled boy as a little cripple exemplifies this attitude. Unlike Western concepts, Orientals do not attach stigma to this appellation, but consider it a literal description of the individual, the deformity being part of him. This attitude permits the afflicted to view the condition as something to be taken for granted. The disabled is expected to assume responsibilities according to one's capabilities, with more closely aligned family members to lend a hand. This infrastructure is less likely to undermine the family constellation, impoverish the household or necessitate the patient's institutionalization, as is more likely to occur in our society.

Degenerative diseases cause psychic pain to the entire family and are frequently aggravated by physical stress. For example, people with PD often suffer from sleep disturbance which, according to Pollak's findings (1991)) also disrupts the partner's rest. In advanced Parkinsonism the family's anguish may be compounded by dementia and incontinence. A study by Mayeux et al. (1991) showed that a large minority of patients was cognitively impaired and that late onset PD was more likely to be accompanied by dementia. While one may deal with physical symptoms effectively, no equal measures are available for dementia. Such developments elicit feelings of loss of a loved one. Permanent mental changes are likely to disrupt even healthy family relationships. Family interactions change as the condition changes, with some characteristics more prevalent during one disabling stage than another. Where chronic neurological disability exerts long and constant pressure upon family relations, the extensive effects of the chronicity may disrupt already weakened family bonds. Moreover, Stern's study (1993) attested to the presence of depression in 40% of patients with PD; often before the manifestation of motor symptoms. At other times, patients may not be depressed, but family members are, particularly the caregivers for whom professional intervention may be essential to maintain their own mental health and family equilibrium.

The patient who requires twenty-four hour custodial care presents a particular problem. The most frequently cited reason for institutionalization is the triple aggregate of dementia, incontinence and sleep disturbance. Caregivers tend to experience physical and emotional depletion, concomitant with diminution of the family's economic resources. (Younger families with children to support may face an even greater dilemma.) Other pressures are loss of peer and sexual partnership, decreased social status, role reversal, or worse, the triple functions of breadwinner, domestic manager and nurse attendant. Unless the (spouse) caregiver seeks and receives help, excessive demands on the partner's functional capabilities soon undermine one's morale and health. It is advisable to have spouses utilize community and other resources such as suitable custodial supervision for the patient, respite centers, home attendants, assistance from friends and family, etc. Moreover, patients and family members should be encouraged to engage in activities of interest and, most importantly, to participate in support groups. Caregivers need to know that creating time and space for themselves may help them achieve some degree of personal, occupational and/or social freedom. Atwood (1991) advocates support group involvement. It tends to reduce tension and social isolation, afford an opportunity to share feelings and experiences with others in similar situations and to learn effective coping mechanisms. Sometimes institutionalization of the patient is unavoidable and caregivers are plagued by guilt and recrimination. In that case support group participation is of even greater significance.

Where the illness strikes the established family in midlife, issues are of a different flavor. Since there is a greater prevalence of PD among men who are usually the primary breadwinners, their incapacitation, in combination with increased medical expenses, rising cost of living, and lack of self-expression through work may present severe obstacles to other family members. Consequently, when the disability affects the man, the family often suffers financial upheaval.

The man's wife may be the most severely affected family member. If she is active in the work force, she is more likely to be the secondary wage-earner. (Government reports indicate that women's earnings are far less than men's.) Many women are unprepared for changes in the job market, either in terms of skills needed for employment or current work experience. Dyer (1973) found that the labor market was not conducive to middle-aged women's return to work. Their accomplishments and skills may be cruelly denigrated. Women must accommodate to behaviors and attitudes which, too often, are experienced as an assault upon the ego. At the same time, they are assuming responsibilities at home heretofore shared with the husband. This is further complicated by one's own reactions to these new responsibilities often viewed as onerous. Where women assimilate well into the role of primary breadwinner, attitudes in the home may change. This can be experienced by the spouse as devaluation of one's role, particularly in case of an authoritative husband. He may resent relinquishing formerly enjoyed prerogatives. Furthermore, he may refuse to take on duties in the home which he can perform, viewing that, by so doing, he is underscoring his loss of status within the family. Conflicts may arise also from other regions. The whole family may resent the "woman's" absence from home and the perceived or actual reduction in services.

Lesser complications are observed if the disabled member of the household is a woman. A woman's role of homemaker is socially more acceptable, and domestic tasks can be more suitably arranged to coincide with her physical capacities; nor, as Duff et al. (1968) connoted, will the economic effect of her disability be equally consequential to the loss of a man's income. There is also less likelihood of role reversal or change of children's career plans. Generally, a woman's disability in midlife proves only moderately disruptive to family interaction. Life goals have already been established; and children have reached at least chronological maturity. Many such families could and often do create or maintain a socially acceptable lifestyle with some or no outside assistance.

Green (1994) found that family equilibrium during midlife of adult children was more often disturbed by the neurological sequelae of age disabled parents. Socially, the aged couple places less demand upon the family than the single aged individual. The parent's impairment can result in problems of role reversal, with the child becoming parent to the chronological parent. The adult child is expected to take on decision-making responsibilities for the individual upon whom, historically, (s)he had depended, and to take charge for the parent's economic safety and psychological well-being. This at a time when the midlife child looks forward to a period of ease–children have grown and are on their way towards establishing lives of their own, careers have become relatively stable, and generally economic and social goals have been accommodated. It is understandable that the midlife child does not want to take on additional responsibilities. Unfortunately, society and social scientists too often label such feelings as narcissism or at best uncaring. Thought is not given to the individual who must forgo long planned activities or long postponed objectives in order to care for the aged. Marital partners may experience conflict due to divided loyalties, economic limitations imposed upon the family when two households must be financed; and in time spent satisfying obligations not accepted, at least to the same degree by both partners. Feelings of guilt and resentment are not unusual; nor are charges of neglect for compliance with the needs of one member at the expense of another. Too often "needs" of family members diverge or are in opposition. Where the disabled aged member moves into the home of the child, further tension is to be expected. At times, merely, because the household can not accommodate another person; at other times because the new member has no meaningful place in the family and may be viewed as an interloper rather than as a functional family member.

Fortunately, the occurrence of aged parents caring for their adult children with PD is relatively rare. Sprinzeles (1992) found that the most painful experience for the parent was the acceptance of the chronological reversal of this circumstance. It is unnatural and even more difficult for the single parent who has no (close) partner with whom to share one's concerns. However, as cited for other family members, professional help, support groups, community resources, assistance from the family and reduction of social isolation may enable the parent to function and to keep the patient at home.

Siblings are less often in the position of primary caregiving, but may have to assist the primary caregiver. However, most siblings are only tangentially affected by the patient's affliction. Usually, they have established their own lives. In the event of being the principal caregiver, the same guidelines apply to siblings as outlined for other caregivers.

In the final analysis, disability is not limited to the afflicted individual, but impacts on family life. The first step to modification of a problem is identification of its existence. With the cooperation of the involved parties, team approach and holistic medicine positive results can be achieved. Garrett (1952) strongly advocated communication between patient, family and professionals. Also, Strong (1988), based on her own experience, considered support groups invaluable for patients and families to attain better adjustment. The able-bodied family members, particularly the caregivers, need to remember their obligations not only to the patients but also to themselves or a household with one patient will soon have two.

REFERENCES

Atwood, G.W. 1991. "Support Groups: Where You Learn What Your Doctor Hasn't Got the Time to Tell You" *Living Well With Parkinson's Disease.* New York: Wiley and Sons, pp. 149-156.

Buck, P. 1950. *The Child Who Never Grew.* New York: The John Day Co., pp. 1-14.

Duff, R.S., MD, A.B. Hollingshead, PhD, 1968. *Sickness and Society.* New York: Harper and Row.

Dyer, L.D. 1973. "Implications of Job Displacement at Mid-Career." *Industrial Gerontology.* Spring Issue.

Fahn, S., MD, G. Cohen, PhD, 1992. "The Oxidant Stress Hypothesis in Parkinson's Disease: Evidence Supporting It." *Annals of Neurology,* 32(6): 804-812.

Flapan, M., PhD. 1989. "Living with Parkinson's." *PDF Newsletter.* Winter Issue, pp. 3-6.

Garrett, J.F. 1952. "Psychological Aspects of Physical Disability." *Vocational Rehabilitation Series.* No. 210. Washington, DC: Office of Vocational Rehabilitation.

Green, H., PhD. 1994. Personal Communication.

Langston, J.W., W.C. Koller, L.T. Giron 1992. "Etiology of Parkinson's Disease." In C.W. Olanow and A.N. Lieberman, eds. *The Scientific Basis for the Treatment of Parkinson's Disease.* Park Ridge, NJ: The Parthenon Publishing Company, pp. 33-58.

Lipe, H., RN, MN. 1990. "Sexual Function in Married Men with Parkinson's Disease Compared to Sexual Function in Married Men with Arthritis." *Neurology.* 31(9).

Mace, N.L. and P.V. Robins, MD. 1981 *A Family Guide to Caring for Persons with Alzheimer's Disease.* New York: Warren Brooks Edition, pp. 211-216.

Pollack, C.P., MD and D. Perlick, PhD. 1991 "Sleep Problems and Institutionalization of the Elderly." *Journal of Geriatric Psychiatry and Neurology.* 4(4): 204-210.

Stern, Y. and R. Mayeux. 1993. "Mental Dysfunction in Parkinson's Disease." In E.C. Wolters and P. Scheltens, eds. *Mental Dysfunction in Parkinson's Disease.* Vrije Universitiet: The Netherlands, pp. 123-132.

Strauss, A. 1984. *Chronic Illness and the Quality of Life.* Baltimore: C.V. Mosby Co.

Strauss, P.J. 1994 "Medical Coverage for the Middle Class Elderly." *B Section of the New York Times Sunday Edition.* September, 25, pp. 1 and 5.

Strong, M. 1988. *Mainstay.* Boston: Little Brown and Co., pp. 53-55.

Wright, B.A., PhD. 1959. *Psychology and Rehabilitation.* Washington, DC: American Psychological Association.

Yalom, I.D. 1981. *Theory and Practice of Group Psychotherapy.* New York: Basic Books, Inc., pp. 54-89.

Cognitive Change, Dementia and Depression in Parkinson's Disease

Yaakov Stern

Cognitive change is a common manifestation of Parkinson's disease (PD). Specialized tests may be required to detect specific cognitive changes in otherwise functional patients. On the other end of the spectrum, recent studies have noted higher prevalence of dementia in PD than had been previously suspected. Depression is commonly observed in patients with PD, although there is some controversy about whether this is a manifestation of the disease itself, or simply a reaction to the disabling features of the disease.

Depression and dementia can co-exist in PD or depression can precede dementia. In this context, the case history of one patient we have followed is of interest. This 50 year old man had a 10 year history of PD. Sinemet treatment was initiated at age 44 and he responded well. Three years later, he developed depression which was successfully treated with 5-HTP. Three years after this he became significantly functionally and intellectually impaired, and had episodes of confusion, disorientation, agitation and aggression. A biopsy of the right frontal cortex revealed senile plaques, both with and without amyloid cores and a few neurofibrillary tangles and preliminary analyses suggest that ChAT activity is reduced. This case demonstrates the manifestation of both depression and dementia in a single individual. Wheth-

Yaakov Stern, PhD, is affiliated with the Departments of Neurology and Psychiatry and the Sergievsky Center, Columbia University, College of Physicians and Surgeons, New York, NY.

This work was supported by Federal Grants AGO7370, AGO7232, AGO8702, and the Parkinson's Disease Foundation.

[Haworth co-indexing entry note]: "Cognitive Change, Dementia and Depression in Parkinson's Disease." Stern, Yaakov. Co-published simultaneously in *Loss, Grief & Care* (The Haworth Press, Inc.) Vol. 8, No. 3/4, 2000, pp. 143-149; and: *Parkinson's Disease and Quality of Life* (ed: Côté et al.) The Haworth Press, Inc., 2000, pp. 143-149. Single or multiple copies of this article are available for a fee from The Haworth Document Delivery Service [1-800-342-9678, 9:00 a.m. - 5:00 p.m. (EST). E-mail address: getinfo@haworthpressinc.com].

er the depression was an early sign of the biological changes associated with AD or represented an independent manifestation of PD is unclear.

DEPRESSION IN PD

Three forms of depression are most often reported: major depression, dysthymic disorder, and atypical depression with anxiety.[1-3] Major depression is a chronic dysphoric mood associated with changes in appetite, sleep, concentration, and accompanied by psychomotor retardation. Dysthymic disorder is a similar but intermittent mood disturbance with periods of relatively normal mood.[4] Atypical depression, accompanied by intermittent anxiety has recently been described.[3] The use of well defined diagnostic criteria for depression, such as those in DSM-III-R,[4] is crucial to ensure that diagnosis is as reliable as possible.

Depression of moderate to mild intensity is most frequently reported, and has been most frequently investigated. As many as 40% of patients with PD will become depressed during their illness with 25% of these patients experiencing depression prior to the onset of overt motor manifestation of PD or within a year of their onset. Dooneief et al.[5] estimated the prevalence of depression in PD to be about 47%, while the incidence was about 1.9 % annually. The cumulative risk was about 1.8% per year. In some cases, depression can be associated with mild intellectual dysfunction[6] and even frank dementia.[7]

Some investigators argue that because PD and primary depression share some clinical manifestations, the resultant higher frequency of mood alterations might be expected. A relationship between the severity of depression and the severity of physical manifestations has been inconsistently observed, which would favor this concept.[8] Also, patients with equally physically disabling disorders are often found to be depressed. For example, one study found patients with rheumatoid arthritis to be as depressed as those with PD because of the similar degree of impairment in functional activities of daily life.[8]

On the other hand, Santamaria et al.[9] reported the onset of depression prior to, or just after, the onset of PD. This would occur at a time when, presumably, the motor manifestations of PD are minimal, suggesting that biological changes may occur which predispose to a mood disorder. Also, many investigators have not found an association between the severity of motor manifestations of PD and depression. Finally, depression has been associated with serotonergic changes in PD,[1-2] suggesting that disease-related biochemical changes may predispose to depression.

DEMENTIA IN PD

DSM-III-R[4] criteria for dementia require documented intellectual decline as well as decline in the ability to perform social or occupational function. This functional incapacity must be a result of dementing changes as opposed to physical disability. In PD, it is particularly important to attempt to ascertain the source of difficulty with these behaviors: is the patient incapable of accomplishing them, is there a physical disability that is impeding him, is he too apathetic to carry them out?

The extent to which the dementias of Parkinson's disease (PD) and Alzheimer's disease (AD) overlap remains controversial. As Brown and Marsden[10] point out, some investigators have concluded that the two dementias differ in etiology and phenomenology[11], while, after reviewing the same literature, others remain unconvinced.[10,12,13] Several extensive reviews of comparative studies exist.[13,10-14] While many aspects of memory loss are comparable in demented PD and AD patients, change scores demonstrate a feature of memory loss that is more severe in AD.[15] Thus while dementia in the two diseases is similar in may ways, subtle differences can be detected. Dementia in PD is most likely heterogenous, with some cases due to concomitant AD, some to a "pure" PD dementia, while others due to Lewy body disease.

Although several earlier studies had suggested the prevalence could be as high as 90%,[16] Brown and Marsden[17] argued that those prior investigations had not used criterion-based diagnoses and that as a result most of the estimates were inflated. This was quickly supported by other investigators, who reported prevalence rates between 10 and 16%.[18-21] However, few studies calculated age-specific rates of dementia which might be a better method for investigating prevalence because there is a correlation between age and dementia. In our hospital-based study the prevalence estimate for dementia was 21% in patients whose motor manifestations began after age 70.[21]

A prevalence study of PD with and without dementia an area of Northern Manhattan found that 41.3% of the 179 patients identified in the community were demented.[22] The overall crude prevalence of PD with dementia was 41.1 per 100,000 persons (over age 35: 90.8 per 100,000). The age-specific prevalence of PD-dementia also increased with age, parallel to the increase in PD overall, from 0.5 per 100,000 below age 50 to 787.1 per 100,000 above age 80. The prevalence standardized to the estimated distribution of the 1988 US population, ranged from 5.3 per 100,000 between ages 35 and 64 to 62.5 per 100,000 over age 75. The frequency of PD-dementia was estimated to be less than one-tenth of that for AD.

Mayeux et al.[23] calculated the incidence rate of dementia after nearly 5 years of follow-up of a hospital-based cohort to be 69 per 1000 person-years of follow-up. As age increased, the cumulative incidence, or cumulative risk, of dementia in the cohort also increased. By age 85, the risk of dementia in this cohort had reached over 65%. Rajput et al.[24] found the 5 year cumulative probability of developing dementia in patients with PD to be twice that for age- and sex-matched controls.

These studies suggest that the frequency of dementia is much higher than that previously estimated by prevalence studies. Incidence rates provide a better estimate of the frequency of dementia because it is not affected by mortality. The New York study[23] indicated an incidence rate of 69 per 1000 person years or 6.9%. Compared to standard populations such as the city of Rochester, Minnesota, or a cohort of men in the Baltimore Longitudinal Study, this rate is 6 to 12 times the rate of dementia that would be expected to develop among similarly aged healthy individuals. In terms of the individual patient, this study also indicated that the cumulative risk of dementia was as high as 65% by 85 years of age. Moreover, the likelihood of death is significantly greater for demented patients.

COGNITIVE CHANGES IN NONDEMENTED PATIENTS

Investigators have used PD as a model for studying the role of the basal ganglia in cognition. While the basal ganglia certainly function in many different capacities, Stern[25] suggested a working hypothesis for summarizing behavioral functions of the basal ganglia and in turn the nature of cognitive changes in PD: The basal ganglia are part of a cortico-striatal system that aids in planning and modulating ongoing activity in the absence of external guidance. The cortico-striatal system referred to involves projections from the cortex to the basal ganglia, and some form of feedback returning to the cortex. Prefrontal cortex is probably most involved in this system. The word "activity" is specifically vague in order to encompass behavior ranging from motor control functions to purely intellectual tasks. The tasks share the need for planning and sequencing units of behavior, monitoring ongoing behavior and modifying to continue to meet task demands. This often entails initiating the shift from one unit of behavior to the next when appropriate. Modulating ongoing activity becomes especially important when the environment presents no cues to guide behavior or to indicate whether it is correct. Several categories of cognitive changes noted in early PD are encompassed in this hypothesis, including visuospatial, executive, motor programming and possibly memory changes.

Impairment in various aspects of visuospatial function have been noted in PD.[26-27] These may be a function of patients' inability to plan and conduct motor tasks that require such skills. Difficulties with motor programming have been noted using several paradigms.[28-30] Most studies have not noted a primary deficit in spatial perception, although deficits have been noted on specific non-motor visuospatial tasks.[31]

Executive dysfunction was noted originally on the Wisconsin Card Sort.[32] Similar results have been noted on tasks such as the Odd Man Out, as well as other tasks requiring "set shifting."[33-35] In contrast, there is less consistent evidence for deficit on tasks requiring maintenance of a specific response set.[35]

Some degree of memory loss does appear to be present in nondemented patients with PD,[27] although studies suggest intact ability to register, store and consolidate information. Problems have been noted with delayed response and alternation, recency discrimination, temporal ordering, and dating capacity. It has been suggested that this may in part be related to executive processes such as difficulty organizing strategies for storage or retrieval.[12]

Stern and Langston[36] studied MPTP-induced Parkinsonism, a pure dopamineeficiency syndrome, that occurs without an associated dementia. They found impairment in visuospatial, executive, and verbal fluency tasks all of which require the ability to sequence mental activity. Similar, but less severe, deficits are also found in asymptomatic (for Parkinsonian motor manifestations) patients with limited exposure to MPTP[37] which may imply that there are certain a dopamine-specific behaviors. In contrast, Dubois et al.[38] found than small doses of scopolamine, an anticholinergic, which did not affect memory in healthy elderly produced adverse effects on memory in patients with PD who were not demented. This may suggest that some cognitive changes in nondemented patients are unrelated to dopaminergic depletion.

CONCLUSIONS

Cognitive change, dementia and depression are important features of PD. They complicate treatment of the disease and can be more disabling than the motor features. Careful attention to these aspects of the disease is warranted.

REFERENCES

1. Mayeux R, Stern Y, Cote L, Williams JBW. Altered serotonin metabolism in depressed patients with Parkinson's disease. Neurology 1984; 34:642-646.

2. Mayeux R, Stern Y, Williams JBW. Clinical and biochemical features of depression in Parkinson's disease. Am J Psychiatry 1986; 143:756-759.

3. Schiffer RB, Kurian R, Rubin A, Boer S. Parkinson's disease and depression: evidence for an atypical affective disorder. *Am J Psychiat* 145:1020-2 (1988).

4. American Psychiatric Association, Diagnostic and Statistical Manual of Mental Disorders, Third Edition-Revised, Washington, D.C. 1987.

5. Dooneief G, Mirabello E, Bell K, Marder K, Stern Y, Mayeux R. An estimate of the incidence of depression in idiopathic Parkinson's disease. Arch Neurol 1992; 49: 305-307.

6. Starkstein SE, Bolduc PL, Mayberg HS, Preziosi TJ, Robinson RG. Cognitive impairments and depression in Parkinson's disease: a follow-up study. J Neurol Neurosurg Psychiatry 1990; 53: 597-602.

7. Sano M, Stern Y, Williams J, Cote L, Rosenstein R, Mayeux R. Co-existing dementia and depression in Parkinson's disease. Arch Neurol 1989; 46:1284-1287.

8. Gotham AM, Brown RG, Marsden CD. Depression in Parkinson's disease: a quantitative and qualitative analysis. J Neurol Neurosurg Psychiatr 1986; 49:381-389.

9. Santamaria J, Tolosa E, Valles A. Parkinson's disease with depression: a possible subgroup of idiopathic parkinsonism. Neurology 1986;36:1130-1133.

10. Brown RG, Marsden CD. 'Subcortical dementia': the neuropsychological evidence. Neuroscience 1988;25:363-387.

11. Cummings JL. Subcortical dementia. Neuropsychology, neuropsychiatry and pathophysiology. Br J Psychiat 1986; 149:682-697.

12. Dubois B, Boller F, Pillon B, Agid Y. Cognitive deficits in Parkinson's disease. In Boller R, Grafman J (Eds.) Handbook of Neuropsychology, Vol 5, Elsevier, Amsterdam, 1991:195-240.

13. Whitehouse PJ. The concept of subcortical dementia: another look. Ann Neurol 1986; 19:1-6.

14. Mahler ME, Cummings JL. Alzheimer's disease and the dementia of PD: comparative investigations. Alzheimer Dis Assoc Disord 1990;4:133-149.

15. Helkala EL, Laulumaa V, Soininen H, Riekkinen PJ. Recall and recognition memory in patients with Alzheimer's and Parkinson's diseases. Ann Neurol 1988;24:214-217.

16. Pirozzolo FJ, Hansch EC, Mortimer JA, Webster DO Kuskowski MA. Dementia in Parkinson's disease: A neuropsychological analysis. Brain & Cognition 1982; 1:71-81.

17. Brown RG, Marsden CD. How common is dementia in Parkinson's disease. Lancet 1984;1:1262-5.

18. Lees AJ. Parkinson's disease and dementia. Lancet 1985;1:43-4.

19. Taylor A, Saint-Cyr JA, Lang AE. Dementia Prevalence in Parkinson's disease. Lancet 1985;1:1037.

20. Sutcliffe RLG. Parkinson's disease in the district of the Northhampton Health Authority, United Kingdom. A Study of prevalence and disability. Acta Neurol Scand 1985;72:363-379.

21. Mayeux R, Stern Y, Rosenstein R, Marder K, Hauser WA, Cote L, Fahn S. An estimate of the prevalence of dementia in idiopathic Parkinson's disease. Arch Neurol. 1988; 45: 260-263.

22. Mayeux R, Denaro J, Hemenegildo N, Marder K, Tang MX, Cote LJ, Stern Y. A population-based investigation of Parkinson's disease with and without dementia: Relationship to age and gender. Arch Neurol 1992;49:492-497.

23. Mayeux R, Chen J, Mirabello E, Marder K, Bell K, Dooneief G, Stern Y. An estimate of the incidence of dementia in patients with idiopathic Parkinson's disease. Neurology 1990; 40: 1513-1517.

24. Rajput AH, Offord KP, Beard CM, Kurland LT. A case-control study of smoking habits, dementia, and other illnesses in idiopathic Parkinson's disease. Neurol. 1987;37:226-232.

25. Stern Y. The Basal Ganglia and Intellectual Function. In: Schneider J. (Eds.) Basal Ganglia and Behavior: Sensory Aspects of Motor Functioning. Hans Huber, Toronto, 1987, pp 169-74.

26. Proctor F, Riklan M, Cooper ST, Teuber HL. Judgement of visual and postural vertical by Parking'onian patients. Neurology 1964; 14:287-293.

27. Levin BE, Llabre MM, Weiner WJ. Cognitive impairments associated with early Parkinson's disease. Neurology 1989;39: 557-561.

28. Flowers K. Lack of prediction in the motor behavior of parkinsonism. Brain 1978;101:35-52.

29. Stern Y, Mayeux R, Rosen J, Lison J. Perceptual motor dysfunction in Parkinson's disease: A deficit in sequential and predictive voluntary movement. J. Neurol Neurosurg Psychiatry 1983;46:145-151.

30. Bloxham, C.A., Mindel, T.A., and Frith, C.D., Initiation and execution of predictable and unpredictable movements in Parkinson's disease. Brain, 107 (1984) 371-84.

31. Boller F, Passaflume D, Keefe NC, Rogers K, Morrow L, Kim Y. Visuospatial impairment in Parkinson's disease: role of perceptual and motor factors. Arch Neurol 1984;41:485-490.

32. Bowen FP. Behavioral alterations in patients with basal ganglia lesions. In M. Yahr D (Ed). Basal Ganglia, Raven Press, New York, 1975:169-180.

33. Lees AJ, Smith E. Cognitive deficits in the early stages of Parkinson's disease. Brain 1983; 106: 257-270.

34. Flowers KA, Robertson C. The effect of Parkinson's disease on the ability to maintain a mental set. J Neurol Neurosurg Psychiatry 1985;48:517-529.

35. Richards M, Cote LJ, Stern Y. Executive function in Parkinson's disease: set-shifting or set maintenance? J Clin Exp Neuropsych 1993; 1 5:266-279.

36. Stern Y, Langston W. Intellectual changes in patients with MPTP-induced parkinsonism. Neurology 1985; 35: 1506-1509.

37. Stern Y, Tetrud JW, Martin WRW et al. Cognitive change following MPTP exposure. Neurology 1990; 40: 261-264.

38. Dubois B, Danze F, Pillon B et al. Cholinergic-dependent cognitive deficits in Parkinson's disease. Ann Neurol 1987; 22: 26-30.

Speech-Language Therapy
for Patients with Parkinson's Disease

Celia Stewart

Speech disorders like decreased loudness, imprecise articulation, and acceleration of words at the end of sentences are common symptoms in patients with Parkinson's disease. The decreased loudness associated with Parkinsonism is often related to respiratory muscle involvement and reduced expiratory drive. The air is presented to the glottis in an inefficient manner resulting in ineffective vocal fold vibration, decreased voice loudness, and a rough voice quality. Speech is imprecise due to stiffness, bradykinesia, and hypokinesia of the oral facial muscles. Speech-language therapy can be effective in ameliorating the symptoms of the dysarthria and improving independence and quality of life.

Approximately 89% (Logemann, Fisher, Boshes, and Blondsky, 1978) of the patients with Idiopathic Parkinsonism, also known as Parkinson's disease (PD), have a speech disorder called hypokinetic dysarthria. According to Mutch, Strudwick, Roy, and Downie, 1986, only 4.4% of the people who have Parkinson's disease have seen a speech pathologist. The discrepancy in the number of patients referred for therapy and the number with speech problems probably reflects a lack of awareness of the gains that can be made in speech-language therapy.

The dysarthria associated with Parkinson's disease can be mild and intermittent or so severe that communication is restricted or interrupted. Fluctuations in severity also occur in response to medications and fatigue. Some patients' lives are restricted by the communicative disorder, because they are

Celia Stewart, PhD, is Assistant Professor, Department of Speech-Language, Pathology and Audiology, New York University, New York, NY and Adjunct Instructor, Mount Sinai Medical Center, Department of Neurology, New York, NY.

[Haworth co-indexing entry note]: "Speech-Language Therapy for Patients with Parkinson's Disease." Stewart, Celia. Co-published simultaneously in *Loss, Grief & Care* (The Haworth Press, Inc.) Vol. 8, No. 3/4, 2000, pp. 151-155; and: *Parkinson's Disease and Quality of Life* (ed: Côté et al.) The Haworth Press, Inc., 2000, pp. 151-155. Single or multiple copies of this article are available for a fee from The Haworth Document Delivery Service [1-800-342-9678, 9:00 a.m. - 5:00 p.m. (EST). E-mail address: getinfo@haworthpressinc.com].

151

forced to quit their jobs because of their speech and because, socially, they listen rather than talk. These changes can lead to isolation.

The speech disorder usually begins as a mild reduction in voice loudness or as increased voice roughness. The change can be so mild that the patient and his family are unaware of the difference in his speech. As time goes on, the speech disorder gradually worsens and the patient's family becomes aware that it is hard to understand the patient's speech, that the patient does not talk as much, or that his/her friends avoid calling. The patient is asked to repeat his/her speech and he becomes irritated and wonders why people do not pay attention and listen when he talks. Talking becomes effortful and frustrating for the patient and his/her family until talking finally becomes limited.

The speech disorder, hypokinetic dysarthria, is characterized as decreased voice loudness with monopitch, monoloudness, and prosodic insufficiency (Darley, Aronson, and Brown, 1975, and Brin, Fahn, Blitzer, Ramig, Stewart, 1992). "The shades of inflection to emphasize a point disappear, the volume of the voice is reduced, pronunciation of consonants is defective and the sentence often ends in a mumble" (Selby, 1968, p. 188). Decreased voice loudness has been identified as one of the first signs of Parkinsonism and one of the symptoms that responds well to speech therapy (Ramig, 1993, Ramig, 1994). Increasing speech loudness increases speech intelligibility. When a patient's voice is loud enough, his speech is easier to understand.

Some patients have disfluent speech and repeat words, phrases, and sentences. A few patients will "exhibit a progressive acceleration of words towards the end of a sentence, similar to the festination of gait" (Selby, 1968, p. 188). Other symptoms include imprecise consonants, inappropriate silences, short rushes of speech, and variable rate (Darley, Aronson, and Brown, 1975). When the words are produced with rapid repetitions and decreased loudness, speech intelligibility is decreased and communication is impaired.

Communication can also be impaired when patients with Parkinson's disease lose spontaneous movements such as gestures and facial expression. If a patient does not smile, nod, or wave when he sees and talks with an old friend, the friend may misunderstand the intention and meaning of the speech and think the patient is angry, bored, or disinterested. The friend may start to avoid the patient or may stop initiating greetings or conversations with the patient. As a result, the patient becomes isolated. When non-verbal communication is restricted, it may be easier for the patient to sit passively and listen rather than to speak. The patient may experience frustration with speech and may shake his head and seldom talk.

Patients who receive treatment for dysarthria have improvement in their speech intelligibility and patients who do not receive speech therapy do not improve (Johnson and Pring, 1990, Robertson and Thompson, 1984 and Scott and Caird, 1983). Speech gains appear to last for at least three months following the end of therapy (Johnson and Pring, 1990, Robertson and Thompson, 1984 and Scott and Caird, 1983). Speech therapy can focus on several parts of the speech production system including increasing loudness, respiration, articulation, and resonation. It is important to choose the type of therapy that will be most helpful to the patient so that maximum gains can be attained.

Oral facial muscle stiffness, bradykinesia, and hypokinesia (Caligiuri, 1987, Denny-Brown, 1962, Gath and Yahr, 1988, Hunker, Abbs, and Barlow 1982) and decreased motor coordination (Connor, Abbs, Cole and Gracco, 1989) have been described as symptoms that accompany dysarthria in patients with Parkinson's disease. Speech-language therapy can focus on oral exercises to increase the accuracy, range and coordination of motion of the articulators. Consonants and vowels are produced by making specific sequences of movements of the articulators. If the movements are imprecise, if the articulators do not reach their targets, or if the movements are not coordinated the speech sounds will be altered and speech intelligibility will be reduced. Therefore, increasing the range and accuracy of motion of the articulators can improve precision of articulation and overall speech intelligibility.

Therapy that focuses on increasing the loudness of speech is more effective and has a longer lasting effect than therapy that only focuses on oral exercises and respiration (Ramig, 1993, Ramig, 1994). Not only do patients respond better during therapy but the gains were maintained for three to six months following the cessation of therapy (Ramig, 1993, Ramig and Bonitani, 1991, Ramig, 1994). Increasing the loudness of speech appears to coordinate the movements of respiration, phonation, and articulation, thereby increasing speech intelligibility. "In working with a patient with Parkinsonism, a tape recorder is used constantly. It permits the patient to compare the volume of his voice with that of the therapist and to adjust his volume accordingly. In many instances this is all that is necessary, for most patients are unaware of their weakened voices until they hear them from a source outside themselves and are able to evaluate comparative loudness levels more accurately" (Hoberman, 1958). Once a patient has learned to speak louder, the improvement can usually be maintained (Ramig, 1994).

Speech amplification by an electronics device has been viewed as a simple solution to a difficult problem. If decreased speech loudness is the only symptom, amplification can be helpful. However, if the speech is unclear due to a combination of decreased loudness, "lack of rhythm and inflection and slurred articulation . . . , little benefit may be gained from amplification" (Greene and Watson, 1968). Even with the advances in miniaturization of amplification, making the speech louder mechanically will not compensate for the other elements of dysarthria that frequently occur in patients with Parkinson's disease. Therefore, amplification alone is rarely effective, but can work well in combination with speech therapy.

The power of our speech comes from the air we breathe. When we breathe, our chest wall expands and our diaphragm descends and flattens. Breathing exercises have been directed at improving the excursion of the respiratory muscles. The loudness of speech is supported by adequate expiratory drive. If expiratory drive is reduced the loudness of speech, length of phrases, and precision of consonants is reduced. When we have upright posture, our chest wall has more room to expand and our diaphragm has more room to descend. If posture is slumped forward, chest wall expansion and diaphragm movement is reduced. When patients have good posture their speech can be supported by adequate expiratory drive, but if the posture is slumped, expiratory drive is reduced. Therefore, increasing the general overall posture through increasing the patients level of activity and by having the patient in physical therapy (Palmer, Mortimer, Webster, Bistevins and Dickinson, 1986) can improve posture and endurance and reinforce the goals in speech-language therapy.

Some patients who have Parkinson's disease report having difficulty recalling words in conversational speech. The pauses that occur when the patient stops to recall words lead to hesitations and pauses in their speech. This decreased verbal fluency may be related to aging or may be a symptom of Parkinson's disease (Gurd and Ward, 1989, Hanley, Dewick, Davis, Playfer, Turnbull, 1990, Scott and Caird, 1984). Regardless of the origin of the disorder, speech-language therapy can facilitate word retrieval by having patients recall words in categories or by making word associations. When words are easier to recall, the patient will be able to focus on the motor aspects of speech and speak more loudly and more clearly.

In light of the fact that current research shows benefits from speech therapy, the number of referrals for therapy should increase over the 4.4% reported in 1986. Although studies of efficacy of treatment are seldom beyond criticism, the number of studies indicating benefit from therapy encourages physicians to refer patients for rehabilitation. Speech-language therapy can help patients maintain independence and improve their quality of life.

REFERENCES

Brin M.F., Fahn S., Blitzer A., Ramig L.O., Stewart C.F. (1992). Movement disorders of the larynx. In Blitzer A, Brin MF, Fahn S, Sasaki CT, and Harris K. (Eds.). *Neurological Disorders of the Larynx* New York: Thieme Medical Publishing.

Caligiuri, M.P. (1987). Labial kinematics during speech in patients with Parkinsonian rigidity. *Brain 110*, 1033-1044.

Connor, N.P., Abbs, J.H., Cole, K.J., and Gracco, V.L. (1989). Parkinsonian deficits in serial multiarticulate movements for speech. *Brain 112*, 997-1009.

Darley F.L., Aronson A.E., and Brown J.R. (1975). *Motor Speech Disorders.* Philadelphia: W.B.Saunders.

Denny-Brown D. (1962). *The Basal Ganglia and their Relation to Disorders of Movement.* London: Oxford University Press.

Gath, I. and Yair, E., (1988). Analysis of vocal tract parameters in Parkinsonian speech. *Journal of Acoustical Society of America. 84*(5) 1628-1634.

Greene, C.L. and Watson, B.W., (1968). The value of speech amplification in Parkinson's disease patients. *Folia Phoniatrica, 20,* 250-257.

Gurd, J.M., and Ward, C.D. (1989). Retrieval from semantic and letter-initial categories in patients with Parkinson's disease. *Neuropsychologia 27,* 734-746.

Hanley, J.R., Dewick, H.C., Davis, A.D.M., Playfer, J., Turnbull, C. (1990). Verbal fluency in Parkinson's disease. *Neuropsychologia, 28*(7), 737-741.

Hoberman, S.G. (1958). Speech techniques in aphasia and Parkinsonism. *Journal of Michigan State Medical Society. 57,* 1720-1723.

Hunker, C.J. Abbs, J.H. and Barlow, S.M. (1982). The relationship between Parkinsonian rigidity and hypokinesia in the orofacial system: a quantitative analysis. *Neurology, 32,* 749-754.

Johnson, J.A., and Pring, TR. (1090). Speech therapy and Parkinson's disease: a review and further data. *British Journal of Disorders of Communication 25,* 183-194.

Logemann, J.A., Fisher, H.B., Boshes, B., and Blondsky, E.R., (1978). Frequency and cooccurrence of vocal tract dysfunctions in the speech of a large sample of Parkinson patients. *Journal of Speech and Hearing Research.* 47-57.

Mutch, W.J., Strudwich, A.R., Roy, S.K., Downie, A.S., (1986). Parkinson's disease: disability, review and management. *British Medical Journal, 293,* 675-677.

Palmer, S.S., Mortimer, J.A., Webster, D.D., Bistevins, R., and Dickinson, G.L., (1986). Exercise therapy for Parkinson's disease. *Archives of Physical Medicine Rehabilitation, 67,* 741-745.

Ramig, L.O., (1994). Speech therapy for patients with Parkinson's disease. In Koller, W. and Paulson, G. (eds.) *Therapy of Parkinson's Disease.* Marcel Dekker: New York.

Ramig, L.O., (1993). Therapy for patients with Parkinson's disease. *NCVS-Status and Progress Report-5,* 83-90.

Ramig, L.O., and Bonitati, C.M., (1991). The efficacy of voice therapy for patients with Parkinson's disease. *NCVS-Status and Progress Report-1,* 61-86.

Robertson, S.J. and Thompson, F. (1984). Speech therapy in Parkinson's disease: a study of the efficacy and long term effects of intensive treatment. *British Journal of Disorders of Communication 19,* 213-224.

Scott, S.A., and Caird, F.I., (1983). Speech therapy for Parkinson's disease. *Journal of Neurology, Neurosurgery, and Psychiatry. 46,* 140-144.

Scott, S.A., and Caird, F.I., (1984). The response of the apparent receptive speech disorder of Parkinson's disease to speech therapy. *Journal of Neurology, Neurosurgery, and Psychiatry. 47,* 302-304.

Selby, G. (1968). Parkinson's disease. In Vinken, P.J. and Bruyn G.W. (eds.) *Handbook of Clinical Neurology. Volume 6,* Chapter 6. Amsterdam: North Holland Publishing.

GI Problems in Parkinsonism

Joseph C. Sweeting

This paper discusses what is certainly the most common symptom in patients with Parkinsonism, mainly constipation, as well as another common problem, dysphagia or difficulty in swallowing. It was interesting to learn that Dr. Parkinson himself noted as far back as 1817 that many of the patients he was describing were constipated, so this is a problem with a long history in back of it. Starting at the top of the GI tract, dysphagia will be discussed first. Dysphagia means difficulty in swallowing and there is a long list of possible causes for dysphagia. Patients with Parkinsonism usually have this symptom because of an inability to coordinate muscular contraction in the pharynx and upper esophagus in order to propel food down the esophagus and into the stomach. In order to investigate this problem a barium swallow can be obtained. Xrays are taken as barium passes through the mouth to the stomach. This sometimes is a rather bizarre experience for patients with Parkinsonism. The patient is asked to lie on a table, a straw is put in his/her mouth and the table is tilted back and forth while the patient tries to swallow. Sometimes the patient is tilted upside down. Swallowing under such conditions is virtually impossible for many Parkinsonian patients. The xrays obtained are of little value. If the physician and radiologists work together, however, it is possible to replicate the home situation to some extent and obtain some useful information. This usually means taking xrays of the patient sitting erect and being given adequate time to initiate the swallowing.

Although dysphagia may be caused by problems in the esophagus itself, patients with Parkinsonism usually have a problem centered in the pharynx

---

Joseph C. Sweeting, MD, is Professor of Clinical Medicine, College of Physicians and Surgeons, Columbia University, New York, NY 10032.

[Haworth co-indexing entry note]: "GI Problems in Parkinsonism." Sweeting, Joseph C. Co-published simultaneously in *Loss, Grief & Care* (The Haworth Press, Inc.) Vol. 8, No. 3/4, 2000, pp. 157-159; and: *Parkinson's Disease and Quality of Life* (ed: Côté et al.) The Haworth Press, Inc., 2000, pp. 157-159. Single or multiple copies of this article are available for a fee from The Haworth Document Delivery Service [1-800-342-9678, 9:00 a.m. - 5:00 p.m. (EST). E-mail address: getinfo@haworthpressinc.com].

and hypo-pharynx, or even in the mouth. These patients have little saliva, particularly if they are on certain drugs which tend to decrease salivary flow and they have real difficulty in manipulating their tongue so that it is difficult to propel a bolus of food from the pharynx into the esophagus. As a result of this inability to initiate a strong muscular contraction, food can easily pass inadvertently into the trachea, or windpipe, rather than the esophagus. It is then aspirated into the lungs causing possible aspiration pneumonia.

On occasions, Parkinsonian patients do get food into the esophagus but can not propel it out. The food must pass down the esophagus largely by the action of gravity. There are certain medications that may help with this process. In the most common type of problem, namely the poor coordination of muscles in the mouth and pharynx, the most helpful therapeutic approach is to enlist the aid of a speech therapist. Speech therapists are people who started out in life primarily focusing on trying to teach people how to speak better when speech deficits are present. Since there is a natural affiliation between speaking and swallowing, it is perhaps not too surprising that speech therapists have been particularly successful in teaching patients how to manipulate their lips, tongues, cheeks, etc., in a way to help move food into the esophagus and hence into the stomach. The type of food that is particularly helpful is often a form of puree or soft food, but not liquids, as might be initially supposed. Liquids pass too easily into the trachea and Parkinsonian patients must take them very cautiously. Soft and pureed foods must be taken very slowly because of the difficulty in sequencing muscle action. These simple approaches will often do far more to help the Parkinsonian patients with eating than any drugs prescribed by the physician.

If it is determined that the problem is primarily in the esophagus, there are some medications that have proven to be useful. These are mostly prokinetic agents which help the esophagus to contract more efficiently. There are several of these on the market. The most recent one to be introduced is cisapride, which does add to the propulsive action of both the esophagus and the stomach. This is fortunate since another digestive problem that is experienced by many Parkinsonian patients is a delayed emptying of the stomach. Normally about half the food that enters the stomach should leave it within two hours. In situations of delayed gastric emptying, food may remain for as long as 8-12 hours. On occasion when a gastroscopy (a fiberoptic examination of the stomach) is performed to look for an ulcer or some other form of pathology, pills that have been ingested as long as 24 hours before may be found. This lack of effective emptying of the stomach may have a significant bearing on the availability of a variety of medications since almost all drugs are active only when they are absorbed from the small intestine beyond the stomach. It is possible to determine the effectiveness of gastric emptying by performing a gastric emptying study. This employs a small amount of radioactive material that is added to food and the rate which the tracer leaves the stomach can be determined with an external counter. If there really is a significant delay in the passage of medications from the stomach, this may account from some of the on-off phenomena that are so common in Parkinsonian patients. Prokinetic agents may be helpful in alleviating this.

The constipation which is such a problem for Parkinsonian patients is basically due to poor contraction of the colon. It is not entirely clear why this occurs. One theory focuses on a degeneration of nerve endings in the colon, particularly in the AuerbachMeisner Plexus which is where connections of nerve cells occur in the wall of the intestine. When these nerve endings disintegrate for any reason, the colon may lose its ability to contract. There is also some thought that Parkinsonism itself may itself directly involve the colon. There have been reports of finding material known as Lewy bodies in the colon. These are usually confined to the brain in Parkinsonism. The management of the constipation is never easy. Some patients become quite distended and develop colonic impactions. This may lead to leakage of fluid around the impaction causing something that almost appears to be a diarrhea. This can lead to the inappropriate use of agents to further slow the bowel. It is sometimes necessary to obtain an xray of the abdomen to determine if there is a large amount of stool present. When the constipation or impaction is severe, the patient will require a variety of treatments. Any laxatives that are given should be in the form of liquids such as Citrate of Magnesia. The agents that are commonly employed for other types of constipation such as Senekot, ExLax, etc., are often not appropriate for patients with Parkinsonism. Bran and other forms of fiber that can be very useful for some types of constipation, may simply cause more impaction with Parkinsonism and must be used with caution. In recent years the use of an agent called lactulose has found favor in this situation. It contains the type of material that is not absorbed as it passes through the upper intestine. Therefore it brings a large amount of fluid in the form of osmotic diarrhea. When it reaches the colon, bacteria turn it into acids which help to evacuate the colon. Some patients with Parkinsonism may need to be on Lactulose on a regular basis. The prokinetic agents such as cisapride that are helpful in promoting contraction of the esophagus and stomach may also have some modest effect on the colon, although by themselves they are rarely adequate to prevent constipation. Patients who are prone to constipation need careful observation by their families and physicians because this common problem can often escalate into a major medical, or even surgical, emergency. With proper management the problem can usually, although not always, be controlled.

Self-Care:
The Parkinsonian's Wellness Map

Arlene Teichberg

INTRODUCTION

Unlike the common cold which arrives then departs suddenly leaving little or no traces behind, Parkinson's disease (PD) is a chronic, progressive neurological disorder with a slow, insidious onset. By the time physical symptoms manifest, extensive destruction of the nerve cells in the part of the brain called the substantia nigra has already occurred. Since dopamine is produced in the substantia nigra, the lack of this important chemical results in the inability of the nervous system to receive and transmit messages which control bodily movement. To date, many treatment approaches exist; but there is no cure (Duvoisin 1991, Lieberman, Gopinathan, Neophytides, and Goldstein n.d.). While a technical discussion of PD symptomatology is beyond the scope of this paper, general symptoms of PD are familiar and feared, such as rigidity, tremor, bradykinesia (delay in starting and slowness of all movements), and difficulty with handwriting, balance and walking. (Lieberman et al., ibid.: 5-6). People diagnosed with PD may become terrified and depressed as they envision a life of downward decline, eventual helplessness and dependency, and an inability to complete lifelong dreams.

Major challenges face those who live with chronic, degenerative, and/or life threatening diseases. Effective patient self-care, subsumed within the larger concept of optimal management of PD (and other serious illnesses), requires patient and family to address many of the complex situations noted

Arlene Teichberg, PhD, CSW-R, is Director, Service Advocacy for Families and the Elderly (Senior Connections) and a Psychotherapist (Private Practice), Congers, NY.

[Haworth co-indexing entry note]: "Self-Care: The Parkinsonian's Wellness Map." Teichberg, Arlene. Co-published simultaneously in *Loss, Grief & Care* (The Haworth Press, Inc.) Vol. 8, No. 3/4, 2000, pp. 161-168; and: *Parkinson's Disease and Quality of Life* (ed: Côté et al.) The Haworth Press, Inc., 2000, pp. 161-168. Single or multiple copies of this article are available for a fee from The Haworth Document Delivery Service [1-800-342-9678, 9:00 a.m. - 5:00 p.m. (EST). E-mail address: getinfo@haworthpressinc.com].

here as well as others which may arise: (1) overcoming denial and accepting the reality of the diagnosis; (2) finding a doctor one trusts and with whom one can be an informed, active partner as well as patient; (3) learning about available treatment techniques and adaptive/assistive resources; (4) facing and making necessary career/retirement decisions; (5) financial planning and knowledge of entitlement programs; (6) finding and participating in self-help support groups. Clearly, major illness requires that patient and family obtain needed services and also begin an orderly process of life planning.

Paradoxically, the person who thought s/he was an unfortunate victim, inherits both the challenges of illness and the opportunities for creating a blueprint for healthy living–for his/her personal wellness map. The foreshortening of time left for life has often changed peoples' perspectives intensifying their pleasure with daily living, enhancing personal relationships, taking time, in short, to see the sky, to smell the daisies. This paper identifies and explores some important aspects of patient self-care which promote an enhanced sense of wellness: (1) the positive self and the power of positive thinking; (2) maintaining good physical self-care; and (3) promoting health through mind/body interactions.

THE POWER OF POSITIVE THINKING: DEVELOPING A POSITIVE SELF

The negative transformation of one's body through disease or other physical trauma causes affected individuals to become frightened of who and/or what they have become. In chronic, progressive illnesses symptoms worsen, so that many affected individuals feel they cannot trust their bodies to perform consistently. Bodily integrity is compromised, as is self-image. Two Parkinsonians, Sidney Dorros (*Parkinson's: A Patient's View,* 1981) and Jan Peter Stern (*The Parkinson's Challenge: A Beginner's Guide to a Good Life in the Slow Lane,* 1990) have written informative, helpful books which, inadvertently, I believe, convey these authors' fear and negative self-images when they are very symptomatic. Over half of Dorros' book deals with his many and progressively worsening symptoms and his medical treatments which became less effective over time. Stern succeeds in scaring his readers when he writes about his tremors, "Unless you have experienced living in a body that at times will not stop shaking, it is hard to imagine the burden which tremors can impose on the challenged person. It can give yourself and others the impression that you are scared or totally out of control" (Stern 1990:16).

Seriously ill persons must battle with negative emotions like depression, resignation, anxiety and fear. Psychopharmacological medications may help. But many ill persons have been helped by searching within themselves for hidden sources of strength or spirituality. Many have been motivated and inspired by examples of people whose bravery, healing experiences and/or self-help capabilities have resulted in better than expected health outcomes. Some people afflicted with chronic, degenerative, and/or life threatening illnesses have written inspirational books about their quests for health in order to share their positive coping strategies and provide hope for others.

What are the intangible emotional qualities of these "successful" patients? While medical rating scales can evaluate the severity of illness symptoms in afflicted individuals, they cannot measure "a patient's initiative, determination, spirit or drive–all qualities which can transcend the patient's disability" (Lieberman, ibid.: 15). Authors who have coped successfully with serious illness address themes relevant for most patients such as: a search for excellent medical treatment; informed, caring doctors who work in partnership with their patients; a search for quality of life; understanding and valuing loving relationships with family, friends, and colleagues; and developing ways of living which promote maximum mental and physical health (Cousins 1984, Cousins 1979, Dorros 1985, Stern 1990). A number of significant insights shared by the authors noted, as well as other practitioners of wellness approaches, include insights that are important guideposts for everyone: the connectedness of mind and body in producing health and illness; patients' ability to learn both about and from their disease and implement new, positive health strategies and lifestyles (Chopra 1990, Chopra 1991, Dossey 1982, Bry 1978, Emery 1977).

Cousins (1979: 69), in a meeting with Dr. Albert Schweitzer was told, "Each patient carries his own doctor inside him. We are at our best when we give the doctor who resides within each patient a chance to go to work." Cousins, who suffered and recovered from several life threatening illnesses– tuberculosis as a pre-teenager, a collagen disorder in his late thirties, and a massive heart attack in his mid-sixties–discovered the power of positive emotions, laughter, self-responsibility in assisting the healing process, and the importance of linking hope and the will to live directly to the body's ability to meet serious threats to it.

Parkinsonians looking for courageous, spirited, and humane role models among fellow PDs may find inspiration in Sidney Dorros' previously cited book, *Parkinson's: A Patient's View* (1981). Diagnosed with Parkinson's at age 36, Dorros recorded his many struggles and triumphs over PD during a twenty year period including reflections on treatment of his PD, on his personality and ambitions, family life, his personal growth through renewed love for his dying first wife, widowhood, new love, and remarriage, and involvement in developing the first PD self-help group in the Washington, D.C. area. Useful psychological insights into and practical information on coping with PD are offered. Dorros identified areas of life, such as work and retirement decisions, where it becomes necessary to accept and accommodate to physical limitations due to progression of PD (see the section entitled, "Accommodation Without Surrender": 129-174). Readers of this book will discover Dorros' innate optimism. He constantly found positives, that is, learning and growth experiences, which emerged from his hardships. A few such examples from his book include: (1) overcoming the traumas of premature retirement through financial planning and saving, taking an early pension and Social Security Disability Insurance; (2) finding that increased personal time was an advantage of retirement, led to reduced stress and fatigue and to more time to develop and follow an improved health regime; (3) reciprocating loving caregiving to his terminally ill first wife despite his severe PD; (4) facing in bereavement his guilt about the emotional and physical hardships his PD had inflicted on his wife; and (5) writing in his book the helpful chapter, "Tips for Coping with Parkinsonism" (Dorros 1981: 177-191).

Many people grow through life challenges. They manifest effective coping strategies and succeed in dealing with all kinds of hardships including serious illness. Positive self-esteem and effective coping skills are essential if Parkinsonians and others with serious, progressive, and/or life threatening diseases are to live with dignity and quality of life. Important components of "positive emotional responses" include: a positive self-image, positive thinking and optimism, determination, initiative, self-responsibility, drive, self-honesty and awareness, the ability to learn from experience, a capacity for both independence and interdependence, a capacity to value, care about, help, praise, and love others, and a willingness to be a contributing partner in one's personal and communal relationships. To be a positive emotional self permits us to both be in our physical bodies and yet, through our emotional commitment to ourselves and others, to become more than the sum of our physical parts.

THE IMPORTANCE OF MAINTAINING PHYSICAL SELF-CARE

Current medical treatment for Parkinson's disease can improve PD symptoms for a number of years, and PD patients today can expect a nearly normal life span. Since PD is a chronic and insidiously degenerative disease, patients who early on take responsibility for being active, educated consumers, rather than passive patients, are in the best position to practice good patient self-care on an on-going basis. Highlighted here are some of the many aspects of good patient physical self-care: (1) compliance with medical and medication treatments as well as with prescribed corrective therapies such physical, occupational, and speech; (2) proper diet; (3) physical exercise; and (4) sufficient rest and sleep.

A broader view of physical self-care also considers the process–the steps, attitudes, and behaviors required to develop, implement and maintain one's good physical self-care as part of one's overall wellness map. The PD patient needs to: (1) find doctors who can communicate and actively work with him/her; (2) educate him/herself about the illness; (3) keep a health history/ medication record; (4) identify, understand, and perform as many aspects of good emotional and physical self-care as possible (some interventions will change as symptoms change); and (5) affiliate with self-help support groups and Parkinson's foundations for emotional support, information on medical advances, peer tips for managing physical activities of daily living and also to support PD research.

Because Parkinsonian symptoms can include rigidity, slowness of movement, difficulty with range of motion and walking, physical exercise is important for PD patients. Exercise (while it does not slow the progression of the disease) helps to: prevent deterioration of muscles from disuse; maintain as much flexibility, strength and coordination as possible; reduce feelings of tension and stress; enhance body tone; improve appetite and rest patterns; and prevent or reduce constipation which is a common problem for Parkinsonian's and for sedentary people in general.

Sidney Dorros (1981) offers a number of practical suggestions regarding physical exercise: (1) keep doing what you like doing for as long as you can–e.g., sailing, camping; (2) consider gentle aerobic activities such as walking and swimming, but don't persist with activities which may cause injury–e.g., give up bicycling if tremors and balance problems lead to falls; (3) consider physical activities that are social and involve other people, such as sports; (4) learn what your body can and can not do, and develop a balanced exercise plan; and (5) develop and maintain regular exercise habits.

While a detailed discussion of exercise and other physical aspects of self-care are beyond the scope of this paper, there is extensive and easily available literature for Parkinsonians and caregivers regarding exercise, physical therapy, safe management of activities of daily living, and use of adaptive/assistive devices to maximize self-care. (Du Pont Pharmaceuticals (1990) offers general advice and basic exercises. Duvoisin (1991: 133-151), Chapter 12, "Common Sense About Exercise." Wichmann (1990) suggests an exercise program for people with PD. Levin (1986) "Roles of Occupational and Physical Therapists," 30-39, and "Helpful Hints," 71-78. Lieberman (n.d.): Chapter 10, "Physical Therapy," 28-31. Robinson (1989) addresses adaptive equipment and activities of daily living.)

PROMOTING HEALTH THROUGH MIND/BODY INTERACTIONS

Never before has there been so much optimism about the possibility of maintaining and even regaining health. A multitude of health and healing philosophies and treatments abound. The numerous proponents of healing through mind/body connectedness range from mystics, faith healers, new age thinkers, to scientific researchers and medical doctors. The person who has a major illness is faced with the existence of and choices between a vast array of traditional medical treatments and non-traditional approaches–the latter ranging from standard medical practices in third world and primitive societies such as shamanism (Achterberg 1985), to "treatments" proclaimed by faith healers and numerous self-styled gurus. Patients are also faced with opportunities to buy all kinds of health food products–which, for the most part, are supplementary to but not in conflict with known and standard medical regimens for their conditions. Our society offers so many health approach options that patient self-care and self-help requires individuals to inform themselves as fully as possible about feasible treatment options and proven outcomes–a large task in this era of information deluge.

In the case of Parkinson's, where no cure is yet known, and in the face of other serious illnesses, it is tempting for patients to throw caution to the winds, to try anything "promising," and to spend great sums of money. In fact, when patients have "tried everything" and still continue to deteriorate, there is danger of severe depression-hopelessness, self-blame, and, possibly, suicide. The challenge for patients and their loved ones is to find approaches which, irrespective of "cure," enhance one's feelings of emotional, spiritual, and physical well being.

Within the last quarter of the twentieth century, the acceleration of interest in mind/body medicine has led to cooperative interdisciplinary practice, research collaboration, and information sharing between scientific researchers, clinical medical practitioners, and professionals in various health, human service, and religious fields. Today, widely used health supporting practices validated by research findings include meditation, biofeedback, stress reduction, and visualization techniques. What these techniques have in common is the use of the mind to "center" the whole person; that is, to reduce inner stress and tension, to image desired, positive states of health and rid oneself of symptoms, feelings, experiences that have caused illness, anxiety, fear, unhappiness. Research has shown that sustained and correct use of these stress reduction techniques has led to some measurable physical health improvements such as lowered blood pressure and reduction of headaches. To begin to delve into the extensive wellness literature, a good starting point is, *The Wellness Book: The Comprehensive Guide to Maintaining Health and Treating Stress-Related Illness,* authored by Herbert Benson, M.D. and Elaine Stuart, R.N. (1992) describes many wellness techniques. This work, which provides an organized source of information about and exercises for using stress reduction techniques, is the product of over twenty-five years of scientific research and clinical practice at Harvard Medical School and three of its major teaching hospitals.

> The Wellness Book combines the best of what you can do to enhance your health and well-being. Our research clinical programs . . . were contributing in a significant fashion to the emerging field of Behavioral Medicine . . . Behavioral medicine is a field that combines the many different disciplines related to the integration of mind and body as it relates to health and illness. It applies this model of health to prevention, diagnosis, treatment, and rehabilitation. This approach to health-care recognizes and respects the contribution of individuals to their own health-care and well being. (Benson and Stuart 1992: xi)

Benson is also the author of *The Relaxation Response* (1975), *The Mind/Body Effect* (1979), and *Beyond the Relaxation Response* (1984). These works deal with ways the mind works with the body to enhance physical health.

CONCLUSION

We have alluded to the many and complex issues which seriously ill persons must address as essential aspects of self-care. The price of not addressing medical, financial, emotional, and relationship issues is too high. However, with every challenge in life comes new opportunities for growth. Parkinsonians, those with other major illnesses, and their loved ones are invited to begin the challenging journey through this new part of their lives where the specter of illness makes its opposites–health, time for what we enjoy, love, purposefulness, and discovery–very precious, to be desired and, hopefully, to be obtained.

REFERENCES

Achterberg, J. 1985. *Imagery in Healing: Shamanism and Modern Medicine.* Boston: New Science Library.
Benson, H. 1975. *The Relaxation Response.* New York: William Morrow.
_____ 1979. *The Mind/Body Effect.* New York: Simon and Schuster.
_____ 1985. *Beyond the Relaxation Response.* New York: Berkley Publishing Company (1st published 1984. New York: New York Times Book Company).
Benson, H. and E.M. Stuart. 1992. *The Wellness Book: The Comprehensive Guide to Maintaining Health and Treating Stress.* New York: Simon & Schuster.
Bry, A. 1978. *Visualization: Directing the Movies of Your Mind.* New York: Harper & Row.

Chopra, D. 1990. *Quantum Healing: Exploring the Frontiers of Mind/Body Medicine.* New York: Bantum Books.

_____ 1991. *Perfect Health: The Complete Mind/Body Guide.* New York: Harmony Books, a division of Crown Publishers.

Cousins, N. 1979. *Anatomy of Illness as Perceived by the Patient: Reflections on Healing and Regeneration.* New York: W.W. Norton & Company.

_____ 1979. *The Healing Heart.* New York: Avon Books (First edition published 1983. New York: W.W. Norton & Company).

Dorros, S. 1985. *Parkinson's: A Patient's View.* New York: Warner Books.

Dossey, L. 1982. *Space, Time, and Medicine.* Boulder, Colorado: Shambala Publications.

Du Pont Pharmaceuticals. 1990. *Living With Parkinson's Disease.* Printed in USA: Du Pont Pharmaceuticals.

Duvoisin, R.C. 1971. *Parkinson's Disease: A Guide for Patient and Family.* Third edition. New York: Raven Press. (First edition published 1978. New York: Raven Press).

Emery, S. 1977. *Actualizations: You Don't Have to Rehearse to Be Yourself.* New York: Doubleday & Company.

Lieberman, A.N., G.Gopinathan, A. Neophytides, and M. Goldstein. No date. *Parkinson's Disease Handbook: A Guide for Patients and their Families.* Staten Island, New York: The American Parkinson Disease Association.

Robinson, M.B. 1989. *Equipment and Suggestions to Help the Patient with Parkinson's Disease in the Activities of Daily Living.* New York: American Parkinson's Disease Association.

Stern, J.P. 1990. *The Parkinson's Challenge: A Beginner's Guide to A Good Life in the Slow Lane.* Third edition, revised. Santa Monica, CA.: DMS Publishers. (First edition 1987).

Wichmann, R. 1990. *Be Active: A Suggested Exercise Program for People with Parkinson's Disease.* Staten Island, New York: The American Parkinson Disease Association.

Using Music Therapy
with Parkinsonians

Concetta Tomaino

For the past fifteen years, I have been a music therapist at Beth Abraham Hospital where I have the privilege of working with Dr. Oliver Sacks. Over the years we have consulted on many cases, the majority of which have been concerning persons with neurologic diseases. Music therapy has proven particularly effective for persons with Parkinson's disease (PD). The affected parts of the brain, in PD, are the basal ganglia. Damage to this area results in problems with sequences and consecutive movement. Music, particularly rhythm, can become a template for organizing a series of movements. This process is not automatic. Music must be particular to the individual and they must be able to "feel" the rhythm. As a music therapist, I explore rhythms with each patient and then incorporate the most effective patterns into the therapy sessions. Patients have reported that by internalizing the rhythmic stimulus they can move, walk, or perform consecutive tasks where previously they froze. In addition, I have made "walking" tapes utilizing the preferable rhythmic patterns. These tapes can easily be used with a portable tape player and turned on whenever needed.

Freezing, difficulties in locomotion, difficulties in the flow of speech, are typical problems in PD which can be helped by music therapy. Some of the goals for music therapy might be to improve walking, moving, synchronizing movements, balance, proprioception, maintaining voice volume, increasing vocal projection, and relaxation. An initial session might consist of vocal and instrumental improvisation, discussion of musical preferences, and playing music, live or recorded, in the preferred genres. Percussion instruments may

Concetta Tomaino, ACMT-BC, is Director of Music Therapy, Beth Abraham Hospital, The Bronx, NY.

[Haworth co-indexing entry note]: "Using Music Therapy with Parkinsonians." Tomaino, Concetta. Co-published simultaneously in *Loss, Grief & Care* (The Haworth Press, Inc.) Vol. 8, No. 3/4, 2000, pp. 169-171; and: *Parkinson's Disease and Quality of Life* (ed: Côté et al.) The Haworth Press, Inc., 2000, pp. 169-171. Single or multiple copies of this article are available for a fee from The Haworth Document Delivery Service [1-800-342-9678, 9:00 a.m. - 5:00 p.m. (EST). E-mail address: getinfo@haworthpressinc.com].

be used to enhance sensation and reinforce symmetry of movement. I worked with a young person with PD who lived independently in the community. For the rhythmic exercises he used a large African slit drum which he played with soft rubber mallets. In describing this exercise he stated "not only do you feel the rhythm but also the resonance of the actual vibration. The feeling is transmitted to your hands, arms and the rest of you. So the combination of the very subtle, vaguely perceivable feel of music combined with the actual hearing of it provides a point of departure or a springboard from which to move."

Music therapy may also be beneficial in enhancing or maintaining vocal projection. Various vocal exercises, similar to those used by singers, can provide techniques for strengthening the voice. Specially programmed musical tapes, as I previously mentioned, can also be used to facilitate every day activities, which are becoming more difficult to perform, e.g,. getting out of bed. Some PD patients have told me that they can lay in bed for an hour before they can get their body to move; however, if they can turn on the tape player or have it turned on automatically, the music will provide the necessary stimulus to get their body moving and out of bed. Another patient stated that he was afraid to go for a walk in the city for fear that he would freeze in the middle of an intersection. He started taking his walkman and tape on his daily outings and turned on the music just before he crossed the street. The music carried him to the other side.

It is important to restate that the music and the rhythm must have a stimulating affect for the individual, not just any music will do. It is also important for the music therapist to find music and or a rhythmic pattern that does reach the patient to the point that the feel of the music can be internalized. The effects of music can be immediate if the person can generate this sort of stimulus for himself, for example, humming a song that has "their rhythm." Although research has shown that a simple metronomic beat can cue walking, in persons with PD, the more the person can internalize and reproduce the music themselves, the more useful a tool it becomes. Counting 1,2,3,4, 1,2,3,4, etc., over and over, for example, may give a person a sense of pulse but it would not necessarily cause him/her to tap his/her foot or move his/her body; yet, add a march or Latin tune to it and a person may notice that he/she is spontaneously moving to the beat.

People have also reported that there are times throughout the day, either between medications or right before they go to bed, when they have too much movement and cannot relax. In these situations, I have made progressive relaxation tapes which may start at a fast tempo to meet the person "where they are at" but then slow down, gradually lulling them to sleep.

These are some clinical examples of how music therapy has proven beneficial for persons with PD. With continued research, we should be able to gain a clearer understanding of why and how music influences motor functioning.

REFERENCES

Sacks, O., Tomaino, C. "Music and Neurologic Disorder," *International Journal of Arts Medicine.* MMB publishers, St. Louis, Vol 1, #1, fall 1991. pp.10-12.

"Music Therapy for Parkinson's Patients," *National Parkinson Foundation, Inc.* 1st Quarter 1992 pp. 10-12. (Interview with C. Tomaino and O. Sacks.)

Accommodating Parkinson's Disease:
A Review of the Perspective
of the Caregiver and the Parkinsonian

Linda M. Waite

INTRODUCTION

Parkinson's disease is a progressively degenerative neurological condition that affects physical, mental and emotional functioning. Caring for a person with Parkinson's disease is a demanding task. Parkinson's caregivers cope with stressors brought on by the Parkinsonian's physical disabilities, dementia, depression, and drug side effects.

Parkinson's disease affects 1 in 100 people over the age of 50 in the United States (Duvoisin, 1984). The prevalence of Parkinson's in the U.S. is estimated to be around 130 people for every 100,000 population (Tanner, 1988). Estimates of the total number of Parkinsonians in the U.S. range from 500,000 (National Institutes of Health, 1983) to one and a half million (Parkinson's Disease Foundation). One in seven people with Parkinson's experience the onset of the disease in their thirties and forties (called young or early onset) (Esibill, 1983). More than 90% of people with Parkinson's disease live at home with their families (Schwab & Doshay, 1981). Given these estimates, it is likely that there are between 450,000 and 1,350,000 in-home Parkinson's caregivers in the U.S. Despite being a population of considerable size, very little is known about Parkinson's caregivers.

Linda M. Waite, MSW, is Parkinson's Disease Foundation Grant Recipient and the daughter of a Parkinson's Disease Caregiver, Hudson, MA.

This review was conducted as part of a larger study (Waite, 1990) supported by grants from the Parkinson's Disease Foundation and the Peninsula Parkinson's Support Group in San Jose, CA.

[Haworth co-indexing entry note]: "Accomodating Parkinson's Disease: A Review of the Perspective of the Caregiver and the Parkinsonian." Waite, Linda M. Co-published simultaneously in *Loss, Grief & Care* (The Haworth Press, Inc.) Vol. 8, No. 3/4, 2000, pp. 173-187; and: *Parkinson's Disease and Quality of Life* (ed: Côté et al.) The Haworth Press, Inc., 2000, pp. 173-187. Single or multiple copies of this article are available for a fee from The Haworth Document Delivery Service [1-800-342-9678, 9:00 a.m. - 5:00 p.m. (EST). E-mail address: getinfo@haworthpressinc.com].

173

As the number of elderly persons in the United States more than doubles in the next 30 years (Doty, Liu, & Wiener, 1985), and as federal funding for elderly and health care programs diminishes, spouses and family members will increasingly be forced to provide care for their mentally or physically ill relatives (Stoller, 1983). Providing this kind of care is extremely demanding (Clark & Rakowski, 1983). This is especially true for Parkinson's caregivers (Waite, 1990), who are often elderly themselves. With the current lack of funding for custodial, in-home, and respite/relief care, many caregivers have no other choice but to depend on their own coping resources. If these services are to be made available, adequate public pressure must be applied. It is important, therefore, that further research into Parkinson's disease and Parkinson's caregiving be conducted, and the information widely distributed.

This review summarizes information on the stages and symptoms of Parkinson's disease; Parkinsonian psychosocial adaptation; stress and coping as it relates to illness; caregiver stress; and Parkinson's caregiving.

STAGES AND SYMPTOMS OF PARKINSON'S DISEASE

Literature on Parkinson's disease is dominated by bio-medical research into the causes of the disease. The description of Parkinson's symptoms as the disease progresses, and their impact on day to day living are presented in this review.

The effect of Parkinson's disease and its drug therapy on the person with Parkinson's is well documented (Goldberg, 1984; National Institutes of Health, 1983; Weiner, 1984; Stern & Lees, 1982; Esibill, 1983). Parkinson's symptoms and drug side effects include restrictions of movement and mobility, diminished independence and sociability, restriction of communication and interpersonal connection, and diminished comfort.

The disease worsens over time. It may begin as a condition that is barely noticeable to friends or associates and progress to a stage of complete invalidism with severe mental limitation. The Physical Therapy Department at Community Hospital and Rehabilitation Center in Los Gatos, California, categorized Parkinson's *physical* symptoms into five stages based on increasing disability and need for assistance. These included "Independent," "Supervision," "Minimal Assistance," "Moderate Assistance," and "Maximum Assistance."

During the "Independent" stage, life for the Parkinsonian and the caregiver can proceed pretty much as it did before diagnosis. Parkinsonians experience loss of locomotion, tremor, poor posture, speech problems, and loss of facial expression. "The characteristic gestures, mannerisms and postures which are so idiosyncratic and personal and essential to speech and communication become sluggish" (Stern & Lees, 1982, p. 7). Parkinsonians at this stage are usually able to drive, to be responsible for their schedule, to pay bills and perform household tasks, to socialize and to work full time. The caregiver can work full time as well.

During the "Supervision" stage, Parkinson's begins to directly affect home life. Parkinsonians experience bradykinesia (slowing of all movements), fatigue, weakness, and lethargy, which reduces their activities. Muscles become rigid which causes ratchet-like movements, and contributes to stiffness, stooped posture when standing and walking, imbalance and the tendency to fall. Parkinsonians might still be able to drive, and may have more fear of being alone. They are able to take care of themselves physically but need reminders from the caregiver, and they may forget aspects of the household routine or bill paying responsibilities. Parkinsonians are less able to clean up after themselves. The Parkinsonian might work part time, and the caregiver can work full time. Having visitors and socializing is still possible, although the Parkinsonian may have difficulty. Socializing depends, in part, on the Parkinsonian's mental limitation. If the mental limitation is "moderate" rather than "none" or "mild," the incidence of socializing is reduced.

During the "Minimal Assistance" stage, the Parkinsonian is probably retired, and the caregiver has dropped to part time employment. Parkinsonians have pronounced difficulties walking, which may include foot dragging, problems with balance, a decrease in the natural arm swing, short, shuffling steps (festination), difficulty starting to walk (start-hesitation), abrupt freezing spells (akinesia) with freezing in the middle of walking (sudden-transient freezing), while turning (turning-freezing), or when about to reach their destination (destination or target-freezing). Parkinsonians have moderate generalized disability, have given up driving, can manage household tasks but need frequent reminders, have difficulty concentrating (they can "get lost"), have communication and eating difficulties, and are not able to socialize.

Socialization is restricted because Parkinsonians may experience drooling, tongue protrusion, excessive sweating, grimacing, an over production of the normal oily coating of the skin (seborrhea), difficulty swallowing (dysphagia) that results in a pooling of food in the throat, coughing or choking to dislodge food that has entered the lungs, and nausea. Anti-parkinson's medications can also cause the person to have hallucinations and paranoid behavior. Parkinsonians also have difficulty beginning to speak, and difficulty speaking clearly. It is difficult for others to understand them because of low voice volume, or a voice that may sound monotonous, breathy, tremulous, high-pitched, hoarse or strident.

By the "Moderate Assistance" stage, caregivers are becoming exhausted. Most are providing 24 hour a day care to a person who needs help tying shoes, shaving, hooking or buttoning clothing, zipping pants, getting into and out of chairs, and turning in bed. Parkinsonians experience significant disability with increased rigidity, increased bradykinesia causing slow and uncertain movements, increased incidence of falling, decreased finger dexterity, and decreased independence in the acts of daily living. Household chores are difficult for them to complete. Communication is severely limited and they have significant trouble eating and swallowing. Parkinsonians are very vulnerable in this state of disability and may not feel safe in the care of anyone other than the caregiver.

During the last stage of the disease, "Maximum Assistance," the provision of care to Parkinsonians is dictated by the strength and stamina of caregivers. The majority of caregivers at this stage are elderly, have usually been providing care for several years, and often have medical problems of their own. Parkinsonians are generally in a stage of complete invalidism with severe bradykinesia and severe rigidity. They are usually bedridden, require the use of a wheelchair, and must be dressed, fed, bathed, etc. If caregivers are not strong enough to move Parkinsonians from bed to wheelchair to bath, or are undergoing medical problems of their own, outside assistance is required.

Throughout the various stages, Parkinsonians and caregivers may have to contend with dramatic fluctuations in motor ability. Called the "on-off" phenomenon (or "yo-yoing"), it can result after several years of drug therapy. The "on" is when the drug is at peak levels, and the "off" is the drop toward the end of a dose of medication. According to Esibill (1983), "This leads to mood swings and variations in alertness and memory, and a person may be transformed from functional to bedridden in a short period" (p. 122). In addition to the "on-off" phenomenon, anti-parkinson's drugs can cause dyskinesia (involuntary movements) at the beginning and end of a drug cycle, or at the peak of the drug cycle.

Throughout the disease, the Parkinsonian's desire or ability to connect superficially or intimately with other people is affected. Reports of dementia, depression, marked anxiety, agitation, memory loss, and confusion are frequent. A lack of desire for sex, fear of being unable to perform satisfactorily, physical inability or discomfort, and the loss of independence in a partnership profoundly impact the sexual intimacy of people with Parkinson's and their caregivers (Esibill, 1983).

Beyond the "Independent" stage, Parkinson's causes great discomfort to the Parkinsonian, which directly impacts on the caregiver. Parkinsonians may experience urinary retention or frequency, burning and cramping sensations, particularly calf cramping with inturning of the toes (dystonic cramps), dizziness or lightheadedness (blood pressure drop) which can be severe enough to cause falling, a slight decline in vision, inability to open the eyelids, burning in the throat or chest, feelings of hot or cold, ankle and foot swelling, dry mouth, constipation, palpitations, hot flashes and flushing of the skin, nightmares, sleepiness (especially after drug therapy), pain in the back and in other muscles, and a change in the sense of taste.

Sleep disturbances are common, and include an inability to fall asleep or remain asleep, and frequent nighttime awakenings, which leave Parkinsonians and caregivers exhausted in the morning. Some people with Parkinson's have a reversed sleep pattern, sleeping throughout the day (napping often), and remaining awake at night.

Because the symptoms of Parkinson's Disease change over the course of the disease, Parkinsonians and caregivers are required to constantly adapt to these changes.

PARKINSONIAN PSYCHOSOCIAL ADAPTATION

According to Dakof and Mendelsohn's (1986) extensive review of the literature on the psychological aspects of Parkinson's Disease, not only has research into the causes and treatment of Parkinson's Disease had a bio-medical focus, but "research on the psychological aspects of Parkinsonism has been focused on disease-related variables rather than on Parkinson patients themselves." They contend that this focus inadequately addresses the ways in which people with Parkinson's and their families strive to overcome and/or adapt to their disabilities and limitations. "We are, for example, largely ignorant of how patients see themselves as having been changed for better or for worse by their illness, the psychological factors that act as buffers against psychological distress, and how the patient's social environment affects and is affected by their illness" (pp. 384-385).

Dakof and Mendelsohn's response to this need was to investigate patterns of adaptation to Parkinson's disease. In an article in *Health Psychology* (1989), they interviewed 44 people with Parkinson's and their spouses about the effects of the disease on their lives. By using the Q-sort technique to analyze the interview data, they identified four clusters of adaptation. These included: Cluster I: Sanguine and Engaged; Cluster II: Depressed and Worried; Cluster III: Depressed and Misunderstood; and Cluster IV: Passive and Resigned. They found that disease severity seemed to be the critical factor that distinguished the patients in Cluster III and IV from those in Clusters I and II. People in Cluster III had more motor deficits, and people in Cluster IV had greater severity of cognitive impairment. The determining difference between Cluster I and II appeared to be attitudinal stance. The factors present in Cluster I but absent in Cluster II were a sense of control, a belief that things could be worse and an ability to put negative thoughts out of mind. Dakof and Mendelsohn (1989) concluded that "Although the present data cannot identify the factors underlying these cognitive differences, premorbid personality and the nature of the couple's marital relationship seem likely candidates" (p. 372).

MacCarthy and Brown (1989) investigated the psychosocial factors of 136 people with Parkinson's using questionnaires that evaluated the clinical severity of the disease, functional disability, depression, positive affect, acceptance of illness, self-esteem, coping, social support, and cognitions relating to the illness. Like Dakof and Mendelsohn (1989), they found the following:

> Psychological adjustment in PD does not straight-forwardly reflect levels of impairment or disability. Instead, it was demonstrated that other factors, particularly self-esteem and coping behavior, help to explain variations in individuals' ability to remain cheerful and adapt to the changes imposed by their illness, independent of their physical state. (p. 48)

They found that three was the median number of "close others" who were potential sources of support, that the availability of social support had little relationship to the process of adjustment, but that instrumental support was a significant predictor of the preservation of well-being. They suggested that satisfaction with support received may have more impact on adjustment than the number of support people available.

MacCarthy and Brown (1989) utilized an adapted form of Folkman and Lazarus'(1980) Ways of Coping Checklist to evaluate coping strategies. They found that people with Parkinson's who limited their coping responses to only helpful strategies fared better than those who tried a wide range of strategies, which included some associated with depression, unhappiness and poor acceptance of illness. "This finding is in keeping with the view that persistent efforts at mastery may be inappropriate or maladaptive in circumstances where the potential for control is limited" (pp. 49-50). The helpful coping strategies used by people with Parkinson's were both problem-focused and emotion-focused, however the strategies that seemed to be associated with poor adjustment were mainly emotion-focused.

STRESS AND COPING AS IT RELATES TO ILLNESS

The cognitive theory of psychological stress and coping was developed primarily by Lazarus and Folkman (Lazarus, 1966; Folkman & Lazarus, 1980; Lazarus & Folkman, 1984; Folkman & Lazarus, 1985; Folkman, Lazarus, Dunkel-Schetter, DeLongis, & Gruen, 1986; Folkman, Lazarus, Gruen, & DeLongis, 1986). According to this theory, stress is a "relationship between the person and the environment that is appraised by the person as taxing or exceeding his or her resources and endangering well-being" (Folkman, Lazarus, Gruen, & DeLongis, 1986, p. 572). Once a person has appraised the person-environment transaction as taxing or exceeding the person's resources, the person utilizes coping, which is the person's cognitive and behavioral efforts to reduce, minimize, master or tolerate internal and external demands. Coping is divided into two major functions, problem-focused coping, which is concerned with dealing with the problem that is causing the distress, and emotion-focused coping, which concentrates on regulating emotion. According to Folkman et al. (1986), "Previous investigations (e.g., Folkman & Lazarus, 1980, 1985) have shown that people use both forms of coping in virtually every type of stressful encounter."

Folkman, Lazarus and Schaefer developed and used The Ways of Coping Checklist to quantify and evaluate stress and coping (Folkman & Lazarus, 1980). The checklist contains 68 items that describe a broad range of behavioral and cognitive coping strategies. The authors classified checklist items into problem-focused and emotion-focused. The checklist is used with a specific stressful event in mind, and participants answer either yes or no to each item. The authors of the Ways of Coping Checklist continue to revise this list to reflect increased knowledge about coping (Folkman & Lazarus, 1985; Folkman, Lazarus, Dunkel-Schetter, DeLongis & Gruen, 1986).

Folkman and Lazarus' problem-focused and emotion-focused categories were also used to classify the coping measure presented by Billings and Moos (1981). They developed a 19 item scale in which participants answered yes or no to each item in response to a recent personal crisis or stressful life event. The items were grouped into three methods of coping, namely, active-cognitive, active-behavioral, and avoidance, in addition to problem-focused and emotion-focused. Billings and Moos (1981) found that their yes/no response format prevented a measure of the frequency or intensity of a coping response. They concluded that "the various categories of coping and a simple count of the number of different coping responses made to an event were only minimally related to the amount of life change required by the event" (p. 153).

The restrictions faced by Billings and Moos were eliminated in the Jalowiec Coping Scale (Jalowiec & Powers, 1981; Jalowiec, Murphy & Powers, 1984). The strength of the Jalowiec Coping Scale, originally a 40 item scale that was later revised to 60 items (Jalowiec, 1988), is that it uses a 5-point Likert format that ranges from "never" to "almost always." In this way, the rate of frequency each coping response is used can be determined. Each of the items were classified as either problem-oriented, which are coping strategies that attempt to deal with the problem or stressful situation itself, and affective-oriented, which are coping strategies that attempt to handle the emotions evoked by the situation. Factor analysis of this scale yielded four categories each with several suggested names. These included: (1) problem-oriented, cognitive, problem-resolving, autonomy-oriented, goal-directed, purposive, or reality-oriented; (2) tension-modulating, avoidant/evasive, morale-maintaining, acquiescent, or palliative; (3) powerlessness, pessimistic, impotency-related, nugatory, or regressive; and (4) other-directed, dependency-oriented, support-related, or linkage-directed.

The above three scales have been used in several studies exploring the relationship between the stressors of a particular illness and coping responses. The illnesses/conditions include hypertension (Jalowiec & Powers, 1981; Powers & Jalowiec, 1987), hemodialysis (Baldree, Murphy, & Powers, 1982; Gurklis & Menke, 1988), myocardial infarction (Nyamathi, 1987), and emergency room patients (Jalowiec & Powers, 1981).

According to Folkman and Lazarus' theory, it can be suggested that Parkinsonians and Parkinson's caregivers experience stress, and would utilize coping responses to manage their stress. To date, the examination of stress, coping and illness has focused almost exclusively on patients. Research quantifying the stress and coping responses used by Parkinson's caregivers has received little attention.

CAREGIVER STRESS

Because Parkinson's Disease causes progressive cognitive impairment and physical disability, Parkinson's caregivers must continually accommodate and cope with changes in both arenas. According to McDowell, Coven, and Eash (1979), the physically disabled experience special problems with self-concept, body image, frustration, anger, dependency and motivation.

Fadden, Bebbington, and Kuipers (1987), in their review of the literature on the burden of caring for the in-home mentally ill, concluded that caregivers may experience restricted social and leisure activities, financial difficulties, particularly if the patient was formerly the breadwinner, anxiety, guilt, feelings of rejection toward the ill person, anger, grief, and a sense of loss. Severe burden in family members was found when the ill person exhibited aggression, delusions, hallucinations, confusion and an incapacity for self-care, most of which are symptoms of anti-parkinson drug side effects or of the disease itself. Additionally, behaviors on the part of the ill person that included lack of communication, affection, interest and initiative, as well as social withdrawal and quiet misery were problematic for family members. The authors concluded that "coping with their relatives' problems frequently results in adverse effects on their own health, both physical and psychological" (p. 291).

Clark and Rakowski (1983), analyzed the caregiving tasks reported in 34 reports from empirical, review and service program sources. They categorized these tasks into three dimensions of caregiving. These included direct care of the impaired family member; (intra)personal tasks, concerns and difficulties of the caregiver; and familial and societal tasks of the caregiver role. Of the 45 items listed in the three categories, 11 were designated as especially stressful or difficult for caregivers, and included: performing activities of daily living for the care-receiver; emotional drain; loss of personal time; gaining knowledge about the disease/condition; drain on physical strength/health; guilt over "negative feelings" toward care-receiver; disappointment or guilt over one's performance; loss/restrictions on future plans and perspective; encroachment on family time; anger at other family members; and interacting with medical, health, and social service professionals.

Poulshock and Deimling (1984) attempted to clarify the concept of caregiving burden by developing and correlating measures for elder impairment, burden, and impact on elder-caregiver-family relationships and impact on caregiver activities. Of the 19 impact measure items that were selected for their factor solution, 8 referred to the loss of personal/social time, 2 referred to conflicts with family, 4 referred to the caregiver's emotions, and 5 to the caregiver-elder's relationship. They found that caregiver depression was associated with both burden and impact. "It is clear from this analysis that caregivers do report feelings of burden and that they are linked both to the impairment that gives rise to them and to changes in objective conditions within the family" (p. 238).

Zarit, Reever, and Bach-Peterson (1980) developed a 29 item self-report burden interview, which they used to investigate how caregiver feelings of burden are affected by the impairment of senile dementia patients and by aspects of the home care situation, including the amount of formal and informal support the caregiver receives. The caregiver indicated the degree of discomfort caused by each item on the burden interview from "not at all" to "extremely." Of the 29 items, 3 referred the loss of personal/social time, 3 referred to conflicts with family, 13 referred to the caregiver's emotions, 7 to the caregiver-spouse's relationship and 3 referred to loss of health or finances. The researchers examined the variables of cognitive impairment, memory and behavior problems, functional abilities and duration of the illness with caregiver burden. They found that the amount of caregiver burden was less when more visits were paid to the dementia patient by other relatives. Unlike other studies, they also found that the severity of behavioral problems was not associated with higher levels of burden.

Baillie, Norbeck and Barnes (1988) investigated the effects of perceived caregiver stress and social support on the psychological distress of family caregivers of the elderly. Perceived stress of caregiving was evaluated using a 16 item, self-report questionnaire with a 5-point Likert scale ranging from "no stress" to "high stress." The items referred to the elder person's behavior, communication ability, emotional or mental state, or relationship with the caregiver; time demands in caregiving; physical or task aspects of caregiving;

effects on other family members; and financial considerations. Satisfaction with social support was evaluated using an 8-item questionnaire with a 5-point Likert scale ranging from "not at all satisfied" to "very satisfied." The items included emotional support, acceptance in caregiver role by family members, contact with others in the social network, and tangible help from others. The authors concluded that caregivers of a mentally impaired elder, "who have been providing care for an extended time, and who have low social support are at high risk for psychological distress or depression" (p. 217).

In an attempt to further quantify caregiver stress and burden, Robinson (1983) developed a Caregiver Strain Index. Robinson considered "stress" and "strain" to be inter-changeable concepts. The index included 13 stressors: inconvenience, confinement, family adjustments, changes in personal plans, competing demands on time, emotional adjustments, upsetting behavior, the patient seeming to be a different person, work adjustments, feelings of being completely overwhelmed, disturbed sleep, physical strain, and financial strain. Respondents could answer either yes or no to each item as it was read by an interviewer. The reliability of the scale was good, with a coefficient alpha for the 13 items of .86.

PARKINSON'S CAREGIVING

Despite the seriousness of Parkinson's disease and its obvious impact on caregivers, very little research has quantified the experiences of Parkinson's caregivers. Dura, Haywood-Niler, and Kiecolt-Glaser (1990), investigated caregiver depression and distress in spouses caring for persons with Parkinson's dementia or with Alzheimer's dementia. They found that both caregiver groups showed greater distress than the control group, and that Alzheimer's caregivers and caregivers for Parkinsonians with dementia did not differ on distress measures. They concluded that both caregiver groups appeared mildly depressed, and that caregiver impairment was strongly associated with the number of daily caregiving hours.

In an unpublished study, Waite (1990) evaluated the stress, coping responses and needs of 206 Parkinson's caregivers using the Jalowiec Coping Scale, the Parkinson's Caregiver Stress Scale, and a Needs Assessment Scale. The latter two scales were developed by the researcher. The results indicated that 22% of the study participants were "very" or "extremely" stressed, and that Parkinson's caregiver stress was strongly correlated to the degree of the Parkinsonian's physical disability and mental limitation. Waite found that 22 coping responses in the 60 item Jalowiec Coping Scale were "sometimes" used and "fairly" helpful, and that coping responses that were Confrontive and Optimistic were most often used and most helpful. Caregivers in this study reported a need for the provision of easily accessible, trustworthy, competent, affordable and/or subsidized services. The utilization of house-hold/domestic help, day care, overnight respite care, and custodial care was consistently less than need, and unmet need appeared to be directly related to a need for financial help.

The research of Dura et al. and Waite is substantiated by Parkinson's caregivers through descriptive reports of their experiences. Parkinson's care-givers must constantly accommodate themselves to changes. The "on-off" phenomenon experienced by Parkinsonians can be experienced by caregivers as "high stress and demand–lower stress and demand." As the disease prog-resses, the world of the Parkinsonian shrinks, which strongly influences the caregiver.

> The range of activities is progressively more restricted. The diversity of contacts and interests gradually diminishes. Attention is focused on fewer and fewer concerns . . . With horizons narrowed, the patient is seeing the world through a peephole. The images may be sharper but the perspective is gone. The mind is still active but the imagination may sometimes run wild. Taken together, these factors can generate fanta-sies that magnify everything including one's previously closely held suspicions, hurts and apprehensions. (Howard, 1987, #3, p. 4)

It is important for Parkinson's caregivers to educate themselves about the effects of the disease and particularly about drug side effects. "Balancing symptomatic relief with side effects requires exquisite fine-tuning, and it is virtually impossible for physicians to know precisely the exact tolerances of each patient" (Howard, 1986, p. 10). Caregivers must be able to discern whether bursts of temper, snide remarks, and recriminations/accusations are an appropriate emotional response to some event in the relationship, or whether these are drug side effects.

Parkinson's caregivers report both similarities and differences between their experiences of caregiving, and those of other caregivers. Howard (1987, #1) described the following aspects of Parkinson caregiving: as the disease progresses, caregiving efforts become "potentially onerous," with commen-surate diversion from other pursuits; worry about the growing backlog of domestic work; frustration; resentment and a sense of deprivation because of curtailed recreational/social activities; social isolation; embitterment; and re-duced willingness to face and deal with Parkinson's on a "day-after-day-af-ter-day" basis without letup.

Some of the reports describe differences. Although Zarit, Reever and Bach-Peterson (1980) found that the amount of caregiver burden was less when more visits were paid to the dementia patient by other relatives, this is often not true for Parkinson's caregivers. Howard (1989) warns against spur-of-the moment visits to people with Parkinson's, even by family members.

> It must be borne in mind that most Parkinsonian patients remain mentally alert even as their physical condition becomes severely impaired. At the same time, they are normally extraordinarily self-conscious about their infirmities . . . Tremors, speech impediment, walking difficulties, all make one not only impatient with oneself, but also often ill-at-ease with others. (p. 6)

For the caregiver, Parkinson's is more than a list of symptoms and drug side effects. It is being vigilant at all times for the sounds of distress–a weak voice calling for help, the sound of the person falling, coughing or choking, something being dropped. It is washing every item of clothing worn by the person with Parkinson's after each day to prevent skin rashes from abnormally oily skin and excessive sweating. It is resigning oneself to the fact that constant cleaning will still not keep up with the particles of food that drop from the Parkinsonian's mouth, or with the trail of viscous drool that marks the passage of the person. It is being awakened every 1-2 hours throughout the night, *every* night, to help the person turn in bed or shuffle to the bathroom. It is making sure medications are taken at the correct times, while at the same time attempting to allow the Parkinsonian to be as independent as possible. It is accepting that dreams must be abandoned, that life must be lived one day or one hour at a time, and that all plans for play, pleasure or social interaction always depend on the moment-by-moment state of the person with Parkinson's. It is somehow learning to cope with the never ending demand for physical strength, and emotional endurance. It is coping with more types and more intensity of stress than most people are ever faced with.

SUMMARY

Parkinson's disease is a particularly demanding condition. It affects both physical and mental capacity, is chronic and is progressively debilitating. As a result, Parkinson's caregivers must continually cope with the changing stressors of the disease. Research has shown that "attitudinal stance" and "psychological adjustment" (i.e., coping) have a significant impact on adaptation to the disease by Parkinsonians. Research with non-Parkinson's caregivers has shown that the negative impact of caregiving on the well-being of the caregiver is quite extensive. These studies have identified several categories of stressors that impact upon caregivers' levels of stress. Several studies have been conducted to evaluate coping responses. Many of these studies researched patients with a specific illness, and the coping responses they used to deal with the stress of the illness. Continuing research into the stress, coping, and needs of Parkinsonians and Parkinson's caregivers is warranted.

REFERENCES

Baillie, V., Norbeck, J. S., & Barnes, L. A. (1988). Stress, social support, and psychological distress of family caregivers of the elderly. *Nursing Research, 37*(4), 217-222.

Baldree, K. S., Murphy, S. P., & Powers, M. J. (1982). Stress identification and coping patterns in patients on hemodialysis. *Nursing Research, 31*(2), 107-112.

Billings, A. G., & Moos, R. H. (1981). The role of coping responses and social resources in attenuating the stress of life events. *Journal of Behavioral Medicine, 4*(2), 139-157.

Clark, N. M. & Rakowski, W. (1983). Family caregivers of older adults: Improving helping skills. *The Gerontologist, 23*(6), 637-642.

Dakof, G. A. & Mendelsohn, G. A. (1986). Parkinson's Disease: The psychological aspects of a chronic illness. *Psychological Bulletin, 99*(3), 375-387.

Dakof, G. A. & Mendelsohn, G. A. (1989). Patterns of adaptation to Parkinson's disease. *Health Psychology, 8*(3), 355-372.

Doty, P., Liu, K., & Wiener, J. (1985). Special report: An overview of long-term care. *Health Care Financing Review, 6*(3), 69-78.

Dura, J. R., Haywood-Niler, E., & Kiecolt-Glaser, J. K. (1990). Spousal caregivers of persons with Alzheimer's and Parkinson's Disease dementia: A preliminary comparison. *The Gerontologist, 30*(3), 332-336.

Duvoisin, R. C. (1984). *Parkinson's disease: A guide for patient and family*(2nd ed.). New York: Raven Press.

Esibill, N. (1983). Impact of Parkinson's disease on sexuality. *Sexuality and Disability, 6*(3/4), 120-125.

Fadden, G., Bebbington, P., & Kuipers, L. (1987). The burden of care: The impact of functional psychiatric illness on the patient's family. *British Journal of Psychiatry, 150*, 285-292.

Folkman, S. & Lazarus, R. S. (1980). An analysis of coping in a middle-aged community sample. *Journal of Health and Social Behavior, 21*, 219-239.

Folkman, S. & Lazarus, R. S. (1985). If it changes it must be a process: A study of emotion and coping during three stages of a college examination. *Journal of Personality and Social Psychology, 48*, 150-170.

Folkman, S., Lazarus, R. S., Dunkel-Schetter, C., DeLongis, A., & Gruen, R. (1986). The dynamics of a stressful encounter: Cognitive appraisal, coping and encounter outcomes. *Journal of Personality and Social Psychology, 50*, 992-1003.

Folkman, S., Lazarus, R. S., Gruen, R. J., & DeLongis, A. (1986). Appraisal, coping, health status, and psychological symptoms. *Journal of Personality and Social Psychology, 50*(3), 571-579.

Goldberg, S. (1984). Independence as a therapeutic goal in Parkinsonism. *Parkinson Report, 2*(2), 6-7.

Gurklis, J. A. & Menke, E. M. (1988). Identification of stressors and use of coping methods in chronic hemodialysis patients. *Nursing Research, 37*(4), 236-248.

Howard, J. L. (1989). How to visit a Parkinson patient. *United Parkinson Foundation Newsletter, 1*, part 1, 4-6.

Howard, J. L. (1987). The little world. *United Parkinson Foundation Newsletter, 3*, part 2, 4-5.

Howard, J. L. (1987). What about the Parkinson partner? *United Parkinson Foundation Newsletter, 1*, part 2, 4-5.

Howard, J. L. (1986). Parkinson's disease and marriage. *United Parkinson Foundation Newsletter, 2*, 10-11.

Jalowiec, A. (1988). Confirmatory factor analysis of the Jalowiec Coping Scale. In C.F. Waltz & O. L. Strickland (Eds.), *Measurement of nursing outcomes. Vol l: Measuring client outcomes* (pp. 287-308). New York: Springer.

Jalowiec, A. & Powers, M. J. (1981). Stress and coping in hypertensive and emergency room patients. *Nursing Research, 30*(1), 10-15.

Jalowiec, A., Murphy, S. P. & Powers, M. J. (1984). Psychometric assessment of the Jalowiec Coping Scale. *Nursing Research, 33*(3), 157-161.

Lazarus, R. S. (1966). *Psychological stress and the coping process.* New York: McGraw-Hill.

Lazarus, R. S., & Folkman, S. (1984). *Stress, appraisal, and coping.* New York: Springer.

MacCarthy, B. & Brown, R. (1989). Psychosocial factors in Parkinson's disease. *British Journal of Clinical Psychology, 28*, 41-52.

McDowell, W. A., Coven, A. B. & Eash, V. C. (1979). The handicapped: Special needs and strategies for counseling. *Personnel and Guidance Journal*, December, 228-232.

National Institutes of Health. (1983). *Parkinson's Disease–Hope through research* (NIH Publication No. 83-139). Bethesda, MD: Author.

Nyamathi, A. M. (1987). The coping responses of female spouses of patients with myocardial infarction. *Heart & Lung, 16*(1), 86-92.

Poulshock, S. W. & Deimling, G. T. (1984). Families caring for elders in residence: Issues in the measurement of burden. *Journal of Gerontology, 39*(2), 230-239.

Powers, M. J., & Jalowiec, A. (1987). Profile of the well-controlled, well-adjusted hypertensive patient. *Nursing Research, 36*(2), 106-110.

Robinson, B. C. (1983). Validation of a caregiver strain index. *Journal of Gerontology, 38*(3), 344-348.

Schwab, R. S., & Doshay, L. J. (1981). *The Parkinson patient at home*(5th ed.). New York: Parkinson's Disease Foundation.

Stern, G., & Lees, A. (1982). *Parkinson's disease: The facts.* New York: Oxford University Press.

Stoller, E. P. (1983). Parental caregiving by adult children. *Journal of Marriage and Family, 45*, 851-858.

Tanner, C. M. (1988). Epidemiology in Parkinson's disease: The search for an environmental cause. *United Parkinson Foundation Newsletter, 4*, Part 2, 5-7.

Waite, L. M. (1990). *Caregiver coping responses to the stressors of Parkinson's Disease.* Unpublished masters thesis, California State University, Sacramento.

Weiner, W. J. (1984). The diagnosis of Parkinson's disease. *Parkinson Report, 2*(2), 5 & 8.

Zarit, S. H., Reever, K. E., & Bach-Peterson, J. (1980). Relatives of the impaired elderly: Correlates of feelings of burden. *The Gerontologist, 20*(6), 649-655.

Medical Expenses and Taxes

Jeffrey S. Wallerstein

The tax laws are constantly changing and the new laws usually seem to be more restrictive on tax deductions. One area in which the Internal Revenue Service (IRS) is fairly generous are medical expenses that may be deducted from one's income. There are two hurdles one must overcome in order to use a medical expense deduction. The following briefly describes the major types of expenses that are deductible, what the hurdles or limits are and where to go for further help. These guidelines are written to be shared with patients.

The first question that comes to mind is: "whose medical expenses can I include?" One can deduct medical expenses for oneself, spouse or dependents. A person generally qualifies as your dependent for medical expense deduction if: (1) that person lives with you for the entire year as a member of your household or is related to you, and; (2) that person is a U.S. citizen or resident of Canada or Mexico for some part of your tax year, and; (3) you provided over half of that person's total support for the calendar year. You may be able to take a person as dependent for medical expenses even though you cannot take an exemption for the person on your tax return because that dependent earned $2,450 or more of gross income or filed a joint return.

You can only deduct medical expenses when you pay for them. It does not matter when you received the service. If you pay by check, the day you mail the check constitutes payment. This is true even if you mailed the check on December 31, 1994 and know your doctor would not receive it until 1995. If you pay by credit card, the date of the charge is considered the date of payment. It does not matter if it takes you two years to pay off the charge. You cannot include medical expenses that were paid by an insurance compa-

Jeffrey S. Wallerstein, CPA, is a member, American Institute of Certified Public Accountants, New York State Society of Certified Public Accountants, Woodbridge, NJ.

[Haworth co-indexing entry note]: "Medical Expenses and Taxes." Wallerstein, Jeffrey S. Co-published simultaneously in *Loss, Grief & Care* (The Haworth Press, Inc.) Vol. 8, No. 3/4, 2000, pp. 189-192; and: *Parkinson's Disease and Quality of Life* (ed: Côté et al.) The Haworth Press, Inc., 2000, pp. 189-192. Single or multiple copies of this article are available for a fee from The Haworth Document Delivery Service [1-800-342-9678, 9:00 a.m. - 5:00 p.m. (EST). E-mail address: getinfo@haworthpressinc.com].

ny or someone else. If you pay $1,000 to your dentist and two months later your insurance company reimburses you $800, you can only take a deduction for $200.

The IRS is fairly generous in what it qualifies as a medical expense. The following table 1-1 lists the major deductible expenses and some examples of non-deductible expenses. Capital expenses for equipment or improvements to your home, if the main purpose is medical care, are deductible. Some types of improvements to your home that would qualify are:

- Constructing entrance or exit ramps to your residence,
- Widening doorways or hallways,
- Installing railing or support bars
- Modifying bathrooms and kitchen cabinets or equipment,
- Modifying fire alarms, smoke detectors and other warning systems.

Only reasonable and necessary costs would be deductible. The costs for upgrading appearances of your property would not be deductible. The cost of the improvement is reduced by the increase in the value of your home. For example, if you installed an elevator in your home for $10,000 the deductible amount would be the $10,000 less the increase in value to your property. If after installing the elevator your property was appraised for $7,000 more the deduction would be limited to $3,000. The $7,000 would be added to the basis of your property. If the capital expense qualifies as a medical expense, the cost of operating and maintaining would be deductible i.e., the cost of electricity to run the elevator and any maintenance.

The cost of medical insurance premiums are deductible under medical expenses. Policies can provide payment for:

- Hospitalization, surgical fees, Xrays, etc.;
- Prescription drugs; or
- Dental care.

The insurance policy can pay you, the patient, or the care provider directly. You cannot deduct premiums you pay for:

- Life insurance premiums,
- Disability insurance
- Policies for loss of life, limb, sight, etc.

The cost of hospital services are deductible. These costs would include lab work, Xray, etc.

Wages and other amounts paid for nursing services are allowable as medical expenses. Services do not have to be performed by a nurse, but just have to be the kind generally performed by a nurse. However, if the nurse provided other services, such as house cleaning, the expense would have to be prorated. Meals provided for the nurse would be a deductible expense.

The amount paid for transportation primarily for and essential to, medical care qualify as a medical expense. Included are: bus, taxi, train, plane fares and ambulance service. For automobile use you have a choice: (1) deduct the actual cost of gas and oil, or (2) use the standard rate of 9 cents a mile. In either case, deduct the actual cost of parking and tolls.

Included in medical expenses is the cost of meals and lodging at a hospital or similar institution if the main reason for being there is to receive medical care. You may be able to deduct the cost of lodging not provided in a hospital while you are away from home. The cost of meals, in this case, are not deductible. The following requirements must be met:

(1) The lodging is primarily for and essential to medical care.
(2) The medical care is provided by a doctor in a licensed hospital.
(3) The lodging is not lavish or extravagant.
(4) There is no significant element of personal pleasure, recreation or vacation in the travel away from home.

If all these requirements, including the personal pleasure part are met, you will be happy to know that the lodging cannot exceed $50 for each night.

In order to support your medical expense deduction, it is necessary to keep receipts and canceled checks evidencing payment. Prepare a permanent record of the name and address of the medical care provider, the date of service and the medical reason for the expense. Without good records it is hard to go back and justify the deductions.

After determining what the total deductible expenses are, you then need to get over two hurdles to actually receive a benefit from the deductions. The first hurdle is, the deductions must be over 7.5% of your adjusted gross income (AGI). The AGI comes from line 31 of Form 1040 and generally is income less certain expenses. For example, if your AGI is $30,000 only medical expenses over $2,500 (30,000 x 7.5%) can be used as a deduction. If your medical deduction was $4,000, only $1,500 would actually be of benefit.

Medical expenses are recorded on the Itemized Deduction Schedule A, lines 1-4. Medical expenses are part of your itemized deductions; therefore, you must be able to "itemize." This means the total of your itemized deductions (mainly medical, taxes, mortgage interest and gifts to charity) must be more than your standard deduction. For 1994, the standard deduction for a single person was $3,800; and married, filed jointly was $6,350. These amounts increase if you are over 65 and or blind. If the total of your itemized deductions is under your standard deduction, you are better off taking the standard deduction. So in this case, even though your medical deductions were over the first 7.5% of AGI you will not receive the benefit of reducing your taxable income since you did not itemize.

Medical expense deductions do not lend themselves to great tax planning techniques. One tip is to bunch your deductions into one year to maximize the potential benefit. A taxpayer may have a choice buying eyeglasses or having a procedure done in this year or put it off until the following year. If the taxpayer already incurred large medical expenses in the current year, and does not anticipate many expenses next year it may pay to have the expense in the current year to clear the hurdles.

A taxpayer can amend prior years' returns to include missed medical deductions. Generally you can amend tax returns for the three prior years.

This manuscript is intended to be an overview on medical deductions. Every taxpayer's circumstances are different, so please consult your tax advisor if you have questions. The IRS does offer some help. To get more information on this topic, call 1-800-TAX-FORM and ask for publication 502 Medical and Dental Expenses. If you still have questions on this topic or any other tax matter, call the same number and ask for the toll-free tax help number in your area. An IRS representative will be available to answer your questions. The representative can also give the location of the nearest Volunteer Income Tax Assistance (VITA) or Tax Counseling for the Elderly (TCE), where *free* tax assistance is available. Walk-in help is also available by Assistors in most IRS offices throughout the country.

Index